Brilliant Breastfeeding

A Sensible Guide

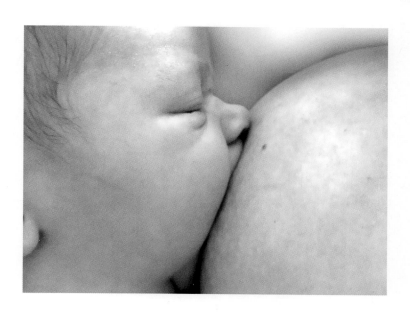

Jo Gilpin

First Published 2018

Cover by Garron Publishing, Adelaide, South Australia
Typeset by Garron Publishing, Adelaide, South Australia

National Library of Australia
Cataloguing-in-Publication entry
Gilpin, Jo
ISBN 978-0-6469924-4-0

Of all the highlights in family life, one of the most exciting and life-changing would have to be the birth or arrival of a new baby. First, second, third, planned or unplanned, it is a most significant time for parents.—— Anonymous

Note from the author

At the time of writing, 'Brilliant Breastfeeding' offers up-to-date breastfeeding and parenting information gained from my many years of first-hand experience and on-the-job observations as a midwife, child health nurse and lactation consultant. However, you should not hesitate to contact a medical practitioner for additional advice, diagnosis or treatment regarding anything to do with a mother's or baby's health issue.

Contents

Introduction

This book is all about making breastfeeding easy, trouble-free and enjoyable. It is factual, interesting, and evidenced-based, aiming to give both parents the very best information to make decisions about feeding their baby. It will help mothers and partners understand how breastfeeding works and how to manage challenges should they arise.

It is for anyone in any country who is expecting or is contemplating parenthood, and ideal for future grandparents to deepen their understanding of how they can support their childbearing family. It is perfect for new parents wanting to take control and enjoy their breastfeeding journey as well as for relatives and friends who can be wonderful supports when they have accurate information.

Worldwide, there is an increase in unnecessary medical interventions during labour and birth. Inductions, epidurals, and caesareans mean that many healthy women with healthy pregnancies do not experience birth naturally. The way baby enters the world can impact on breastfeeding. Considering birthing options and understanding the benefits of quiet skin-to-skin contact with baby as soon as possible after birth, are particularly valuable.

When natural birth is not an option for you, or when medical intervention is necessary, strategies are explained as to how you can maximise the opportunities for a positive start to breastfeeding your baby. This guide will provide practical and non-judgemental ideas to consider. After most birthing situations, encouraging baby's *breast crawl* to his first breastfeed is a beautiful, rewarding and useful experience. It can influence breastfeeding progress.

I write as a mother of three breastfed babies, and also as a Registered Nurse, Midwife, and Child Health Nurse. I have been an International Board Certified Lactation Consultant (IBCLC) for almost 20 years and currently work privately in Adelaide and on Kangaroo Island in South Australia. Throughout my career, I have always been dedicated to helping mothers through a wide variety of difficulties to enjoy and reap the benefits of breastfeeding their babies.

I believe breastfeeding can be made easier with excellent preparation and support.

This is my second book. In 2011 my book called *On the Breast Handbook. Planning for Breastfeeding Success* was printed. It was a source of useful information that led many, mainly Australian mothers, to confident breastfeeding. All copies are sold. *Brilliant Breastfeeding* is an updated version of that book, written with a more global focus because although many women breastfeed with ease, I still see and hear of women all over the world ceasing to breastfeed within the first three months because of obstacles and confusion that could be avoided. It is for those that I am drawn to write more, to expand, to clarify, to simplify and to further encourage and support.

Examining evidence and practical ways to establish breastfeeding successfully is valuable because it helps parents, future parents, and their health supporters to make more informed and confident decisions about the management of birth and feeding practices.

Because breastfeeding isn't always easy, I present all the everyday challenges that, in my experience, can upset breastfeeding goals. These will be tackled by giving you clear and helpful strategies to avoid altogether, to overcome, or seek appropriate help. There is rarely a *problem* that is unresolvable.

The information in this book will help you to have a beautiful start to feeding your new baby no matter how the baby is born. It will encourage you along the way to maintain your nursing relationship for as long as you choose. Weeks, months, years—any length of time spent breastfeeding your baby is valuable. My aim is for you to be empowered, feel confident and truly enjoy breastfeeding your baby or babies.

This book is organised in flowing chapters, starting at the important *before baby is born* time, moving gradually through birth and the first feed, the hospital time, and the early days and weeks. I then progress towards all the aspects that relate directly and indirectly to breastfeeding, as the months go by.

I like to think of 'parents' breastfeeding their baby. Of course, it is the baby who is breastfeeding; the mother breastfeeds her baby, but the father, partner, or other close carers, are of such great importance in giving support, encouragement and love that breastfeeding ideally should be a team effort. And so it is, that sometimes I refer to 'parents' breastfeeding their baby.

Also, I refer to babies as 'he'. This is simply to differentiate between the 'she' of the mother. Not because I prefer boy babies!

Jo Gilpin

Chapter 1

The truth about breastfeeding and breastmilk
Common myths

I believe that breastfeeding is one of the greatest long-term gifts a mother can give a baby and a baby can give a mother. It works both ways. The fact is, there is far more to breastfeeding than the simple transfer of milk.—Jo Gilpin, On the Breast Handbook. Planning for Breastfeeding Success, Hyde Park Press, 2011

If this is your first pregnancy and you are planning to breastfeed your baby, you may well question … What is breastfeeding like? What does it feel like? How does it work? This book may answer some of your queries and help you to get a feeling as to what to expect. If it is your second or subsequent baby, you may want to do things differently; your goals may include aiming for a more extended obstacle-free breastfeeding journey. This information will support you to do just that.

How to describe breastfeeding?

Breastfeeding can be difficult to describe as it is a unique and personal experience between a mother and baby. Perhaps it needs to be experienced before one can fully attempt to express its qualities.

However, many mothers say that it is the firm connection that grows, especially when the breastfeeding relationship flourishes beyond 6 or 12 months, that is exceptionally beautiful and rewarding. Breastfeeding is sometimes easy and sometimes comes with challenges, but overall, it is often described as an absolute highlight of early parenting.

It can be enormously satisfying to give your precious infant the perfect food in just the right amount and at just the right temperature, anywhere, anytime.

The process of producing milk and breastfeeding is helped along by amazing natural body hormones. The main ones are prolactin and oxytocin. They trigger and assist not only the production of milk but the development of strong, loving feelings of connection with your baby. As baby attaches and starts suckling, the many nerves around your nipple area incite the release of these hormones into your bloodstream stimulating the milk to flow. At the same time, these hormones automatically activate the production of more milk to replace what baby drinks.

Hormones are special chemical messengers produced in our bodies by endocrine glands. They control most body functions, including reproduction, emotions and mood. Childbirth and breastfeeding are critically influenced by hormones.

What does breastfeeding feel like?

Each mother would explain it differently, but I would agree with the explanation that when the baby is attached to the breast and is feeding well, it feels like a rhythmic deep drawing sensation or gentle tugging in your breast. During a feed, the suckling changes from being quite a vigorous suck/swallow, suck/swallow at the beginning, to an irregular lighter suckling towards the middle and latter part of the feed. The first week is when your nipples may feel an initial tenderness as they get used to this. However with baby latching correctly this discomfort should dissipate day by day. Baby quickly learns to draw the elastic nipple and surrounding area, *the areola,* deep into his mouth to where his soft palate is at the back of his mouth. This is the ideal position for the very best passage of milk, and in this position, there should be no discomfort at all.

You can feel this area of soft palate by placing a finger towards the back of your own mouth to where the hard palate gives way to a softer part.

When baby first starts feeding, some mothers will feel the sensation of *the letdown reflex* as milk starts to flow. It can be described as a tingly or prickly sensation. This sensation is not usually unpleasant. Breastfeeding should not hurt, especially after the first week. Correct latching or attachment can have such a significant impact on how breastfeeding feels, how the baby gets his food and also on how your milk supply is maintained. Consequently, there is great emphasis on getting attachment right for you in Chapter 5.

I believe one of the very best aspects of breastfeeding your baby, is that you are using your body in the natural way that was always intended. Breasts, no matter what shape or size are there to breastfeed. It is their main job.

By breastfeeding, you are also allowing your baby to use his body the way nature intended. Being so close to you, feeling warm against your skin and able to see you eye to eye, he gains the necessary feelings of safety, security, and love. He is being nurtured in the best possible way. At the same time, he is getting, without a doubt, the ultimate nutrition for his whole body—his heart, kidneys, lungs, gut and brain. He uses all his face and jaw muscles to suckle, creating healthy exercise and precious feelings of connection.

Your breastmilk is a continuation of the perfect food he had in your womb—it is just delivered differently. For approximately nine months all nutrition for growth and development was from your blood that flowed to him via the placenta and umbilical cord. He even had little *tastes* of the food you ate during pregnancy. To continue feeding in this natural way after birth is through the living fluid on the outside—your breastmilk. This continuum of feeding has significant advantages for your body as well as giving your baby the very best of foods. Major long-term health benefits for you both are well researched and documented. (Australian Breastfeeding Association, 2017) Also, breastfeeding is considered the final stage of pregnancy and birth—it makes the cycle complete. Gradually, when baby's milk intake is reducing, as it does when you are weaning, your body naturally resets itself for the possibility of a future pregnancy.

What is in breastmilk that makes it so special?

Breastmilk is unique in that it is the exact composition needed for your baby. It contains perfect proportions of fats, proteins, carbohydrates, vitamins, minerals as well as immune booster cells, enzymes and hormones. It is made from your own body ingredients and miraculously changes according to baby's age, stage of growth and developmental needs. It is perfect for a baby born early or prematurely, or for a six, twelve or eighteen-month-old toddler. Formula, on the other hand, does not change; it stays the same from birth onwards.

Breastmilk contains many hundreds of thousands of unique beneficial bioactive microbes that build up colonies of friendly bacteria in baby's gut. These useful germs aid baby's immune system, protecting against infection and inflammation. They contribute to the baby being healthy and able to reach full developmental potential. (Riordan and Wambach, 2010). This uniqueness cannot be replicated in formula.

How is breastmilk made?

Other aspects of breastfeeding make more sense when you understand how your breasts and body make this wonder-food.

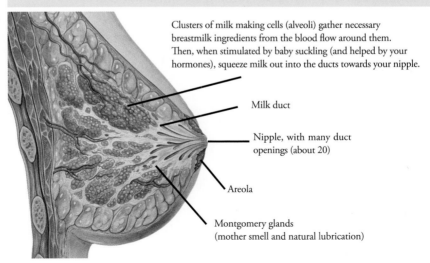

Clusters of milk making cells (alveoli) gather necessary breastmilk ingredients from the blood flow around them. Then, when stimulated by baby suckling (and helped by your hormones), squeeze milk out into the ducts towards your nipple.

Milk duct

Nipple, with many duct openings (about 20)

Areola

Montgomery glands (mother smell and natural lubrication)

The hormones oxytocin and prolactin, play a significant part in breastfeeding. As baby feeds, the many nerves around your nipple area are immediately stimulated sending messages to the pituitary gland in your brain, which automatically releases oxytocin into your blood. This quickly reaches the glandular structures of the breast, stimulating the cells around the alveoli and milk ducts to contract, (the *let down reflex*) resulting in a flow of milk towards your nipples for baby to access for the first part of his feed.

Just as you start breastfeeding and this 'let down reflex' occurs, you may notice that you suddenly feel quite thirsty. This again is related to hormone action. I like to think this is nature's way of reminding you that it is important to care for yourself and keep well hydrated. It is a good idea to have a drink handy when you breastfeed.

As baby suckles and prolactin is released, your breasts are stimulated to gather ingredients from your abundant blood supply to make more milk, replacing the milk taken. It is miraculous, really.

The more often your baby feeds activating these hormones, the more milk your body makes. So there is a constant supply - milk taken by baby is automatically replaced.

Breasts are never really *empty* when you are breastfeeding.

As already mentioned, an essential aspect of your milk production is baby attaching correctly for feeding. If this is not happening, breastfeeding may feel uncomfortable or even painful. The nerves around your nipple area will not receive the right messages for making more milk, and this can lead to worries about your milk supply.

> *Lack of confidence in milk supply—a belief that 'there's not enough milk'—is one of the main reasons mothers often unnecessarily, introduce formula. This can further impact on milk supply and confidence levels, thus affecting successful breastfeeding outcomes. There are many strategies described in Chapter 7 relating to correct attachment and extra stimulation for building your milk supply if necessary.*

How long should you breastfeed?

As the saying goes … how long is a piece of string? And there is no *should*. It is such an individual personal decision between you, your partner, your baby and your particular situation. But finally, it is no one's decision except yours. In some countries, babies are breastfed to four years or more, with mother only gradually weaning as a new sibling comes along. Or, they may continue to breastfeed right through a new pregnancy and *tandem feed* with the new baby. This is completely within normal limits. In western society, the length of lactation is commonly more limited; but there are no rules. Often women say that they would have liked to breastfeed for longer, but due to confusing information, unresolved difficulties, a lack of support or work obligations, the breastfeeding relationship is disappointingly short.

A great guide as you think about breastfeeding goals, is the very sound, evidence-based World Health Organisation (WHO) and the National Health and Medical Research Council (NHMRC) recommendations.

WHO: Since 1948, staff in 150 countries have worked together with governments to build a better, healthier future for people all over the world. Breastfeeding is considered as having a major impact on world health.

NHMRC: Is Australia's leading expert body promoting research and development of health standards affecting public well-being. Evidence supports breastfeeding as the 'backbone of early nutrition'.

They, along with many other health authorities, suggest for babies' best overall development, to 'exclusively breastfeed baby for the first six months, introducing solids around that time, with continued breastfeeding for up to two years of age or beyond'.

Exclusive breastfeeding for six months means that baby receives only breast milk, without additional food or drink, not even water. This is because breastmilk has absolutely everything in it that baby needs: all in perfect proportions for growth and general health. Breastfeeding particularly benefits the baby's brain. Sarah Boseley, a journalist for *The Guardian* paper, reported on a major study of 6000 babies from all backgrounds in Brazil.

It concluded that those babies who were breastfed were more intelligent and spent longer in education than those who were not. The longer they were breastfed, the more they achieved in life. (Sarah Boseley, The Guardian, 2015)

It may sound overwhelming for baby to have only breastmilk for the first six months, but in fact, it can be easily attainable when you settle into a comfortable breastfeeding relationship, purely responding each time to your baby's *cues* or signs that he needs feeding. Each time baby feeds, it gives you an opportunity to rest, relax and admire your baby—all ideal for your own health and well-being.

> *The hormone oxytocin plays a part in this—it is often referred to as 'the wonder hormone' or the 'feel good hormone'. This is because, as well as assisting with breastfeeding, it has the distinct effect of helping you to relax. You may notice this when you settle down comfortably to feed … just as your milk starts flowing and baby is suckling away contentedly … you feel a very gentle … whooooosh of natural relaxant flooding your body, making you feel calm—perhaps even sleepy. This is to be enjoyed.*
>
> *"When mothers breastfeed, both they and the baby secrete comfort hormones called endorphins (morphine-like substances that the body produces) which soothe and calm. Not surprisingly, breastfeeding has been called addictive"* (Chilton 2017)

Are the benefits of breastfeeding proven?

We often hear or read that breastmilk is the best for your baby. But what are the facts? What are the main advantages? Recent research has led to more information to explain these claims. Here are just a few of the reasons why. You may like to follow up on the references to find out more.

For mothers:

Immediately after baby's birth, breastfeeding helps expel your afterbirth or placenta. As baby attaches and starts suckling stimulating the nerves around your nipple, oxytocin is activated, causing your womb to contract to release the afterbirth. This is the very last part of your labour. In the following days after birth, as you feed baby, you may feel discomfort in your pelvic area, somewhat like period pain. This again is the oxytocin causing your womb to contract, reducing blood loss. These *after pains* soon pass. Over the next days, weeks and months, breastfeeding helps tone your womb back into position and then gradually your body back into your pre-baby shape. In the first 12 months after baby's birth, your general weight loss usually occurs steadily and more rapidly than if the baby was formula-fed.

> *People say, 'You're still breastfeeding, that's so generous.' Generous, no! It gives me boobs and it takes my thighs away! It's sort of like natural liposuction. I'd carry on breastfeeding for the rest of my life if I could.*—Actress Helena Bonham Carter

Mother's general health:

The general health benefits for women who breastfeed are significant. There is growing evidence of a reduced risk of cancer, heart disease, diabetes and bones thinning in later life (osteoporosis). The benefits of breastfeeding are dose-related—the longer you breastfeed, the greater the benefits for you and baby. (Davanzo et al., 2016)

For babies:

Breastfeeding gives baby's face, jaw and mouth a fantastic muscle workout. With bottle-feeding, all these muscles are more relaxed; baby's tongue pushes forward to control the flow, and his jaw does not have the same opportunity for exercise.

Naturally, as with any muscles that are used to their full potential, growth and development are superior. It means that breastfed babies have a better chance that teeth will grow straight in a well-shaped jaw. Therefore there is less chance of orthodontic work being needed in later years. (Palmer, 1998)

Growth

In the first two weeks of life, babies who are exclusively breastfed with frequent feeds, usually grow exceptionally well. They regain and pass their birth weight quickly. If this is not the case, or you are in any doubt of baby's progress, do not hesitate to promptly seek assessment by a health professional who you trust.

Breastfeeding, breastmilk and baby's brain.

Babies' brains are only twenty-five per cent formed at birth. They grow rapidly, doubling in weight in the first year. The earliest messages that the brain receives from the close connection and nutrition from breastfeeding and breastmilk can have an enormous impact on children's chances of achievement, success and happiness. (Sears, 2018)

Breastmilk contains all the nutrients that a baby's immature brain needs to achieve its full potential. The first six months is the most vital time for baby's growing brain. The nutrients and the manner in which they work are not fully understood but are thought to be related to the essential fatty acids (linoleic and linolenic) in breastmilk, which are vital for brain, nervous system and eyesight development. There are also many other components that influence optimal development, which are impossible to replicate in formula. There is substantial evidence (Belford, 2016) suggesting that children who are breastfed score higher in tests of intelligence and in the process of acquiring knowledge, reasoning and perception, equating to a higher Intelligence Quota or *IQ*.

Reduced chance of obesity

Obesity in many countries is a serious problem. Reliable evidence is building to show that children who have been breastfed, are less likely ever to be overweight or obese (WHO, 2014).

There are several theories why this is so, but the main ones are firstly, that breastmilk is the ultimate fully balanced food for growth and development. It is a perfect foundation for future healthy food preferences. Secondly, baby never over-feeds; he learns from birth that he is in control of his appetite by only drinking what he needs at each feed. He learns at an early age what *full* feels like. This is partly due to a hormone found only in human milk, called *Leptin*, which helps to regulate appetite and food intake. Baby is less likely to *overeat* when he has access to other foods as he grows. Thirdly, babies who have been breastfed are known to have a reduced risk of chronic diseases that may affect weight, such as Type 2 diabetes, heart disease, atherosclerosis and high blood pressure.

Baby's general health

Breastfeeding and breastmilk have unique qualities that protect baby's health. From early beginnings, when baby has contact with his mother's healthy bacteria or microbiome in her vagina or birth canal, he gains protection from many common infections and viruses. Breastfeeding continues this protection. If mother gets an infection, for example a common cold, baby will immediately receive antibodies through breastmilk to fight the particular germ that is causing the cold. Consequently, babies and children who are breastfed have a reduced risk of respiratory diseases, digestive disorders, ear infections, eczema, meningitis, diabetes and Sudden Infant Death Syndrome (SIDS). Of course, this means many fewer visits to local doctors and hospitals, where antibiotics and other treatment may be needed.

Additionally, looking at the bigger picture, there are huge indirect financial savings to world health systems when chronic diseases are reduced because of women breastfeeding, and babies being breastfed.

Recent conclusions in the new Lancet Series on Breastfeeding are that breastmilk makes the world healthier, smarter and more equal and that the deaths of 823,000 children and 20,000 mothers each year could be averted through universal breastfeeding, along with economic savings of US $300 billion.

What about formula?

Formula as a breastmilk substitute has its place when other feeding options are unavailable, or when you have checked information and have decided that it suits your situation best. However, do be aware, that milk formula companies use very clever marketing strategies to suggest that formula is as good as breastmilk. It is not. How can it possibly be as good? Formula only attempts to imitate breast milk. Most formulas are made from cows' milk and do not contain calcium, fats, protein, vitamins and minerals in the correct form or amounts that baby needs for his exact stage of growth. Additionally, as has occurred in recent history, there is room for error in the manufacturing process, leading to possible contamination. Formula is not perfect for baby's digestive system so is not as easily digested as breastmilk.

However, there definitely are times when breastfeeding, notwithstanding all effort, simply does not work. Mothers can feel a real depth of grief that can colour parenting, possibly even contributing to postnatal depression. I have the utmost respect for these parents and feel their disappointment. Babies do very well with formula when made and used correctly. It is a sensible alternative. Sometimes it is essential for adequate growth, and we are fortunate to have such a backup.

I consider the most critical factor is that babies are truly loved and are nurtured consistently in a loving environment.

Some parents, if it is necessary to consider formula, will seek other options. Well-managed breastmilk banks are being set up in various cities with supplies that can be accessed. While often this donated breastmilk is prioritised for premature and sick babies to give them the best chance for a healthy future, the guidelines do vary.

You may choose to research milk-sharing sites by contacting your state department of health for information in your area. However, there are risks associated with feeding baby breastmilk acquired from individuals or through the internet because the milk may not be screened for diseases or contamination. Generally, there should be processes in place regarding the collection, processing, handling, testing and storing of expressed breastmilk.

Breastfeeding myths—are any of these true?

You may hear, or be told with seeming authority, information about breastfeeding that is actually incorrect. It may stem from those meaning well, but it can cause confusion and loss of confidence. Such advice is unhelpful. The following are just a few common examples of incorrect beliefs. If in doubt about anything you are told, do seek another opinion.

"It helps my partner bond with our baby if I express milk for him to feed."

No, this is not true. There are many better and more helpful ways for partners to connect with their new baby. Cuddling before and after feeds, talking, playing, staying close as you feed all will help with bonding. Besides, it is actually more work to express, wash and store bottles. Suckling at the breast is the best stimulus for making milk and maintaining supply. Mother and baby benefit from the regular stimulation of direct feeding.

"Giving a formula supplement will help my baby sleep."

No, this is not true. Breastfeeding as frequently as he needs, particularly in the late afternoon and evening is the best way to help baby sleep. Unnecessary supplementation can often cause a disappointing downward spiral of breastmilk production and confidence. Milk supply reduces due to less stimulation of baby feeding at the breast. There is the danger that one bottle becomes two bottles, and so your breastfeeding goals become eroded.

"I can't take any medications when I'm breastfeeding."

No, this is not true. There are very few medications that are incompatible with breastfeeding. When mother is unwell and needs to take medication, there will be the tiniest fraction that will be in her milk for a short amount of time. This will not harm baby, and according to Dr Jack Newman in his *Ultimate Breastfeeding Book of Answers,* breastfeeding with a small amount of medication in the milk is not riskier than feeding the baby with formula, except in a few specific situations. If unsure about a particular medicine or drug that you need, do check with a medical officer.

"If I have an occasional alcoholic drink, I cannot breastfeed."

No, this is not true. Many parents wonder about alcohol. Though it is most definitely not a good idea to drink alcohol on a regular basis, an occasional drink will not harm your baby or your milk supply. Again, as with most medications, a small percentage will pass into your breastmilk soon after, but it will pass out again within two to three hours. So if you were planning to have an occasional drink, you could time your breastfeed to just before, during, or several hours after. (Mohrbacher, 2012 and Chilton, 2013)

"Small breasts won't produce enough milk for baby."

No this is not true. All breasts big or small will produce ample milk, providing baby attaches well and removes milk regularly. Larger breasts may have larger storage capacities, so it may mean that there are longer intervals between feeds. Mothers with smaller breasts may feed more often.

"I haven't enough milk for my big baby."

No, this is not true. You will usually have enough milk no matter what his size, as long as his attachment is correct and you feed frequently enough. If in doubt, review the strategies for improving milk supply in Chapter 7.

"My mother couldn't breastfeed, so I doubt that I can do it."

This is not true. In your mother's time, there were probably different attitudes and very little support for breastfeeding. With correct information and support, your superior knowledge will breed confidence and a positive attitude.

It is a huge advantage to have made the decision that you are going to breastfeed your baby before baby is born. This is much better than having an *I will breastfeed if I can, attitude.*

"What I eat affects my milk."

Not usually. Your baby has spent approximately nine months while cosy in your womb, having small tastes of what you have been eating. This happens as your blood containing elements of your diet, courses through the placenta which is attached to your baby. Nothing changes after he is born as he receives the same small traces through your breastmilk. Some mothers do find that if they suddenly eat a lot of one particular thing, for example, cabbage or chocolate, their baby is unsettled, or bowel actions change temporarily.

"I'll wean my baby when he gets teeth."

Not necessary. Teeth usually start appearing around five to eight months and should make no difference to breastfeeding. When baby is attached correctly and feeding, his tongue covers his bottom gums where his first teeth usually appear, so it is not possible for him to bite. However, at the beginning of a feed when waiting for the *let down*, or at the end when he is perhaps playful, he may give you a nip, making you jump. If this occurs, understand that baby did not plan to hurt you. How you react will discourage it happening again. You can calmly say *no* and bring him in closer to you as you try to continue the feed. If it happens again, firmly finish the feed by putting your finger into the side of his mouth to remove him from your breast. He will learn quickly that you mean business and that it is not acceptable for him to do this. As his gums may be irritating him because he is teething, another useful strategy is to push down on his gums with a clean finger before he feeds. Between feeds, a cold teething ring for him to chew on can also soothe his gums and help his teeth to erupt.

Summary

I always respect women's choices on how they birth, feed, and parent— we are all different, do things differently, and really, there are no *rules*. However, I do want to present accurate, up-to-date information, so your choices are knowledgeable, informed, and feel right for you.

I am sure that many of you reading this will have your ideas and understanding about breastfeeding and breastmilk—from your own experience, from what you have heard, or from what you have read. I hope this additional information provides encouragement to help with your decisions.

Chapter 2

Pregnancy
The perfect time to prepare for breastfeeding

To be pregnant is to be vitally alive, thoroughly woman, and distressingly inhabited. Soul and spirit are stretched—along with body—making pregnancy a time of transition, growth, and profound beginnings.—Anne Christian Buchanan and Debra K. Kingsporn, *The Quickening Heart: A Journal for Expectant Mothers.*

Ideally, the time to learn and plan and commit to breastfeeding is before baby's birth. This chapter suggests how to achieve the best start to breastfeeding, no matter how your baby is born.

During pregnancy, there is so much to think about and prepare for, regardless of whether it is your first or subsequent pregnancy. There are many choices and decisions to be made. It can be an exciting but daunting time as aspects of pregnancy and your baby's birth are considered. There is no going back. It is also the perfect time to think carefully about how you are going to feed your newborn. Building your knowledge of breastfeeding will help you gain ideas of what you and your partner want when your baby is born. If you have had a previous disappointing breastfeeding experience, there may be things that you wish to do differently. Knowledge is empowering.

Your breasts are preparing...

Your breasts start preparing for breastfeeding very early in pregnancy. You may notice even before your pregnancy is confirmed that your breasts feel tender and enlarged due to your body's natural hormones *oestrogen, progesterone and others* that stimulate milk duct and breast tissue growth. This growth continues steadily throughout pregnancy until your baby is ready to be born. By six months you will notice that your nipples and areola, *the area around your nipples,* have become darker in colour and small raised spots called Montgomery tubercles are dotted around. These tiny glands help lubricate your nipple area and produce a scent that is attractive to your baby. Additionally, a healthy newborn baby can only see a short distance and is attracted to round shapes like your face and eyes. He is drawn to the dark round shape of the nipples and areolar area. They help guide him towards your breast area and his first feeds.

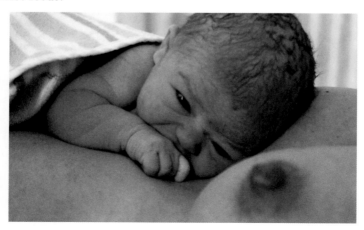

From the middle part of your pregnancy, you will notice that your breasts produce small amounts of a creamy yellow substance. This is colostrum - your first milk. It is sometimes referred to as *liquid gold* because of its vital role when baby is first born. This is normal for your breasts as they prepare for breastfeeding.

It is particularly valuable for baby to receive colostrum. It is very high in protein and antibodies and quickly raises baby's blood sugar and hydration levels after birth. It also acts as a laxative to help baby pass his first bowel action. In doing so, he is less likely to be jaundiced. Colostrum also helps baby's digestive tract to develop well by introducing useful, friendly bacteria, which are advantageous to his immune system.

Sometimes it is suggested that this colostrum is expressed and collected before baby is born. It can be reserved and deep frozen in the unlikely event of baby needing complementary feeding after birth. Having this saved colostrum would reduce the need for baby to have anything other than breastmilk in the early days after birth.

It is wise to discuss this with your midwives and medical staff if you are considering the antenatal expression of colostrum.

With skin-to-skin contact and allowing baby to suckle within the first hours after birth, the need for supplementation with anything other than breastmilk - except in extreme cases should be unnecessary.

Following evidenced-based research, it is now formally acknowledged that women who are diabetic or have diabetes that has developed during pregnancy (gestational diabetes) can safely express breastmilk in late pregnancy without causing harm to their babies.

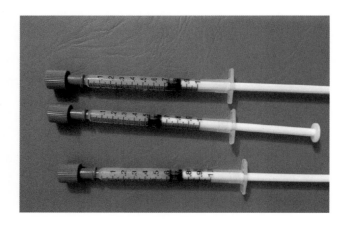

In the photograph, these three 1ml syringes contain expressed colostrum that a second-time mother expressed in the last two months of her pregnancy. This mother chose to do so because of what she experienced with her first baby. She had had an induced start to her labour, an epidural to manage pain, and was separated from her baby after the birth while he was assessed by medical staff. Consequently, he missed the opportunity to have immediate close skin contact. When he was returned to her, firmly bundled in wraps hours later, he was sleepy and slow to learn to attach and suckle. He then lost weight. Although some weight loss is very normal after birth, hospital staff considered it over the acceptable amount and gave him formula in a bottle. If she had stored colostrum, even this small amount as above, formula would not have been needed. Unfortunately, this scenario is common in hospitals around the world.

This can also apply to any mother in a healthy pregnancy who wishes to express and freeze some colostrum to take to the hospital at the time of confinement. Babies will be less likely to receive formula in the first twenty-four hours of life. (Forster et al., 2017)

There are additional benefits of expressing colostrum before baby is born for the *just in case* situation. It is useful to learn how to express. While doing so, you become more familiar with handling your breasts and with how they work. The following strategies can be used if you choose to express colostrum during the last months of pregnancy. (Pearson-Glaze, 2018).

Firstly, try experimenting by briefly practising expression while showering, letting the drops of colostrum wash away. More on hand expression is included in Chapter 7.

- Have a small clean container such as a medicine cup ready and ideally some syringes bought from a pharmacy, as illustrated

- Be warm and relaxed, with well-washed hands

- Massage breasts gently to help the colostrum flow

- Hand express from both breasts, taking care not to cause pain or discomfort. *Hand expression is best because of the minimal amounts that you are aiming to collect. Remember, in the first few days, your baby will only have very small feeds of approximately five mls per feed*

- Begin with two to five minutes of expressing on each side, two to three times a day

- The colostrum will flow very slowly, so let it drip into your container

- It can be drawn up and collected in the syringe, then refrigerated

- You can add collections together in one syringe in one day, as long as the syringe is refrigerated between collections

- Once you have expressed for the last time for the day, clearly label and date, before placing in the freezer

- When you have gathered several in the freezer, put together in a ziplock bag ready to take to the hospital in a cooler-pack when your baby's birth is imminent

- Once at the hospital, ensure they are again stored in a freezer—it may be advisable for your birth partner to know where they are

If for any reason you and your baby are separated at birth, or unable to breastfeed, your colostrum can be defrosted as needed. If your baby needs supplementary nutrition, your colostrum can be used.

Your body is preparing

Towards the latter part of your pregnancy, you may find that you wake more than usual in the night. This may be to pass urine, or because you are aware of baby's movements or that you are uncomfortable with aches and pains. However, this could also be nature's way of preparing you to wake for night feeds after the baby is born. The aches you feel in your body are most probably due to the hormones acting on your joints, increasing their flexibility to allow baby to pass through your birth canal more easily.

Your womb practices contractions towards the end of pregnancy. These are felt as painless tightenings called *Braxton-Hicks* contractions. They help thin and soften the cervix muscle at the lower end of your womb, ready for baby to pass through.

Also fascinating, are the changes in the birth canal particularly towards the end of pregnancy. There is a flourishing growth of millions of friendly and useful bacteria, which is like a climax to the body's preparation for baby's entry into the world.

Rarely discussed with parents and future parents, is the significant value to baby's overall health when he has access to this supply of beneficial bacteria or good germs as he passes through the birth canal.

How do you learn about breastfeeding? What can you do?

Opportunities to explore breastfeeding come in many ways. Knowing how you learn best can help. For example, you might like to read to understand, or watch, listen and ask questions. There are high-quality books that can be found in most libraries and good bookshops. Antenatal classes are helpful, and often there is a specific session on baby feeding. Talk to other people about breastfeeding, for example, your doctor, midwives, friends, your mother, aunts, etc. As you learn, make a list of support people and organisations that may be useful after your baby is born.

Include your partner and support people

A helpful way to prepare for a positive breastfeeding experience is to involve your partner or support person(s) as much as possible. I mentioned in the introduction how beneficial fathers or partners are in supporting breastfeeding mothers. They can be vital. Knowledge of how breastfeeding works and why it is so valuable often results in a naturally encouraging attitude and helps breastfeeding and parenting become more of a *team effort*. During pregnancy is the perfect time to discuss baby feeding, so you will both be committed and involved together when learning opportunities arise.

Resource list

As you progress through your pregnancy, gather together what you think might be useful information. In this way, you can build a personal *resource list*. Difficulties can arise with breastfeeding, and knowing where to go quickly for help can reduce concerns enormously. Often small problems or queries can be instantly solved, leaving you able to enjoy your baby with more confidence. It can be stressful to start searching for the right help when you are tired and have a new baby. You may never need this list, but it will be invaluable if you do.

Your *resource list* might include virtually any contact, phone number, email address or website that you think might be interesting or helpful.

Possible ideas might be:

- 24-hour breastfeeding hotline contact number

- My local child health centre, address and contact number

- Hospital or birthing unit contact details

- My doctor or medical clinic's details

- Midwife contacts, if having a home birth

- Doula (birthing companion) contacts, if having one

- Local lactation consultants (find by googling 'Find a Lactation Consultant' or FALC)

- Personal contacts; friends, relatives and acquaintances - preferably ones who have successfully breastfed their babies and whom you feel comfortable talking with.

After birth feeding plan

Often *birth plans* are discussed during pregnancy. The birth of your baby is a crucial momentous event. However, on average, the delivery is over within hours before other significant activities take over, one of which is the vital aspect of feeding.

Even though there is a degree of unknown about your baby's arrival, it is a positive step to have an *after birth feeding plan*. With this, you, your birthing partners and medical staff will be clear as to what you would like to happen after your baby is born.

Thankfully it is now more commonly acknowledged by midwives and medical staff that the time immediately after birth can play a vital role as to how breastfeeding proceeds. Babies who attach and feed within one hour of birth have more chance of breastfeeding successfully.

> *According to statistics, babies who feed in this early post-birth time are often breastfed for a longer duration. Ultimately, these babies and their mothers receive physical and emotional health benefits from the more sustained breastfeeding experience.* (Minchin, 1988)

An *after birth feeding plan* will enable you to be clear about what you personally would like to happen to help get breastfeeding off to the best start. You can use some, or all of this plan and adapt it to almost any birth situation.

Here is a suggested plan for you to consider, with reasons for the suggestions.

- I would like my baby placed on my abdomen straight after birth.

  Skin-to-skin or tummy-to-tummy contact enhances baby's instincts and reflexes that are particularly heightened immediately after birth. It is the best way to keep baby warm and is a calming reward after the birth. Parents can look, feel, and enjoy baby for the first time.

- Please allow at least an hour of uninterrupted skin-to-skin time after my baby's birth. I would like to watch him *crawl* or wriggle to my breast to attach by himself for his first feed.

  This often takes an hour or more, and naturally lays the foundation for correct attachment for feeding—it's almost as if a good latch is imprinted in baby's brain. This will help with subsequent feeds.

  As a lactation consultant, I often work with women with breastfeeding concerns that possibly began because their baby did not have the opportunity for quiet, uninterrupted skin-to-skin time leading to the first breastfeed. This aspect is often not talked about, and consequently many women and their partners do not realise the enormous value of babies breastfeeding in this first hour after birth. This time is sometimes called 'The Magical Hour.'

  Just knowing about it is exceptionally valuable; it helps to give you the information and the confidence to discuss it with your caregivers. Then, you can expect that no matter how your baby is born, he will be given the opportunity to have this precious experience as soon as is possible after birth.

- If there are necessary procedures could they be done later, or while my baby is resting on my chest?

  I do not want to be separated from my baby.

- I want to avoid washing my breast area for twenty-four hours and delay baby's first bath until after he is feeding well.

  I want both of us to keep our familiar birth smells that will help subsequent breastfeeds.

- I will be flexible, in the case of my needing, or choosing medical intervention during my labour and birth. I will use some or all of our *after birth feeding plan* to suit our particular birth situation.

- I do not want my baby to have a dummy or pacifier.

  Pacifiers can cause 'nipple confusion' in the early weeks of breastfeeding. Sucking on a silicon teat is very different to suckling at breast.

- I wish to breastfeed exclusively.

  I do not want my baby to have any formula.

- My partner (or support person) will advocate and speak for me if necessary.

  We are in this together.

  This after birth feeding plan can be discussed with those you are involved with during pregnancy—for example, family, midwives and doctors. This will help to make it clear as to what you would ideally like to happen when your baby is born.

Summary

As you progress through pregnancy, learn as much as you can and gather a *resource list* of contacts you think might be handy. Involve your partner or support person as much as possible. Make a firm decision as to how you want to feed your baby with a clear *after birth feeding plan* to help everyone involved know your intent.

Chapter 3

How can a natural birth help breastfeeding?
Ideas for other birth situations

The experience of birth is vast. It is a diverse tapestry woven by cultural customs, shaped by personal choices, affected by biological factors, marked by political circumstances. Yet the nature of birth itself prevails in the elegant design of simple complexity.—Harriette Hartigan

To fully utilise your *after birth feeding plan* and have a positive start to breastfeeding, it is an advantage for you to know how a natural birth can help you.

After a natural birth, baby is usually awake and alert. His primary senses of sight, hearing, touch, taste and smell are heightened. He is ready to meet you for the first time, hear your voice, feel your warmth and climb towards your breasts.

Even though you may aim for an intervention free birth, it is not always possible. By being flexible and aware of your options, you can, to a great extent be the leader in how you birth and start your breastfeeding experience, in any birth situation.

This chapter explains the advantages of natural birth and the best ways to maximise the beginnings of breastfeeding.

It is normal for babies to be born naturally. By natural birth, I mean one that is started by contractions that are driven by your own hormones or chemical messengers. This happens spontaneously when your baby is ready to be born—usually, around your expected date of delivery, give or take a week or two around 40 weeks. The hormones do a fantastic job of loosening your body to allow baby to come down through your vagina or birth canal. These hormones help you manage pain and discomfort. When baby is passing through into the lower part of the birth canal, there is a surge of these hormones that help you cope and bear down for your baby's birth. At the time of this hormonal peak, some mothers describe feelings of intense exhilaration.

Ideally, breastfeeding baby within an hour after birth is best because baby uses his natural instincts and reflexes to find and attach to the breast to suckle. Already mentioned is the importance of baby latching correctly for breastfeeding success. The first breastfeed is the ideal time for optimal attachment to be learnt. Breasts are soft before your mature milk has arrived. Baby is usually ready for suckling and is looking for the round, darker shape of your nipple area. He is enticed by colostrum smells. This is the perfect time to begin to lay the foundations of trouble-free latching.

Why do interventions during labour sometimes interfere with breastfeeding?

The involvement of induction to start labour, intravenous therapy with medication to hurry it along and epidurals to reduce pain and discomfort, often result in holding up the beginning of breastfeeding. This is because the natural chain of events for birth are interrupted. The medication used for an epidural means the baby during labour gets a dose of it as well, possibly contributing to him being less alert when born. Newborn reflexes for crawling towards your breast may be dulled.

With an epidural, there is also a higher risk of a slower second stage of labour (because of the block in the sensations of impending birth), and therefore a possible need for forceps to help baby out. This means that there is more chance that he is separated from you after birth while staff ensure his breathing and heart rate are satisfactory. This, in turn, means he may not have immediate skin-to-skin time, missing the opportunity to be breastfed within the first hour.

It is not uncommon if you have an epidural to actually end up having a caesarean for baby's birth, which may be disappointing. (Goer, 2017). This is major surgery, and again has its set of difficulties relating to separation from you and the early breastfeeding start. One thing can lead to another, like a cascade of interventions, and often little is explained to parents. Recent research suggests that birth intervention may be linked to an increased risk of long-term health problems in children. (Dahlen, 2018).

Birth is sometimes considered to be *just got through somehow* or *endured* rather than as an advantageous journey for you and your baby to take. How much thought or explanation is given regarding the benefits to you both to have a vaginal birth? Is your healthy body encouraged and supported to do what nature intended?

In Australia, at this point in time, 30 per cent of all births in public hospitals and 43 per cent of births in private hospitals are by caesarean section. Many countries have even higher rates of intervention, China having one of the highest at around 50 per cent.

Because of this rapid increase in unnecessary inductions and caesarean rates, the World Health Organisation (WHO) has made official recommendations that no country in the world should need an induction rate over 10%, or a caesarean rate higher than 10-15%. They should only be performed when medically necessary. These recommendation are in an attempt to kerb this escalating problem. (WHO, 2016)

By having a natural birth, baby has the advantage of collecting his mother's genetic and bacterial data as he passes through the birth canal. This carries valuable information. Additionally, it is like a priceless boost of probiotics and prebiotics in his system. It *kick starts* his immune and digestive systems. Immediately, he has a degree of protection from harmful germs and a boost to his immune system. This is extremely useful. (Porteus, 2014)

As mentioned earlier, mothers' normal vaginal flora (or microbiota) increases dramatically during pregnancy. This is quite normal and happens for a reason. The rich medium of beneficial bacteria is nature's way of preparing the birth canal for baby to pass through during labour. As he does, he is literally bathed in these microorganisms which prime, or 'jump start' his immature immune system. A healthy immune system is vital for digestion, prevention of infection and inflammation. The immune system quickly develops as a result of this microbiota, and antibodies are produced to fight any harmful bacteria. Babies that are born this way get the largest exposure to these millions of healthy 'uniquely mother' bacteria. These natural bacteria are further encouraged through breastfeeding and breastmilk. Mouth to skin contact as baby breastfeeds also transfers bacteria from mother's skin to baby's gut. This is all significant as recent research suggests that lack of access to mother's microbiome could influence aspects of future health.

What about babies born by caesarean?

Understanding how healthy immune systems evolve, gives you the powerful knowledge to make decisions. Although sometimes caesarean sections are vital for medical reasons, it does mean that babies born this way are not exposed to their mother's birth canal and therefore are not bathed in her microbiome. The bacterial mix is different and comes from other first contacts, like the medical staff's hands and the operating room. There is a lower level of good bacteria, which can hinder digestion and can negatively impact on the developing immune system.

Seeding baby's immune system

Because there is much positive evidence emerging about this, it would not be unreasonable to discuss with caregivers the possibility of having a swab placed in your vagina while caesarean surgery is taking place. (Randle, 2015) This can be removed and rubbed all over baby after birth—skin, eyes, mouth, nose. Perhaps the father or partner can do this. Baby will then receive the advantage of mother's microbiome. This is called 'seeding' baby's immune system.

Additionally, passage through the birth canal results in baby's lungs being cleared of the fluid that was in and around him while in your womb. The natural compression makes his airways ready for his first breath and welcome cry.

Because medical procedures during labour are so common in all countries, how can you sensibly aim for a natural vaginal birth, while at the same time appreciating the vital backup of medical and surgical support if it is essential?

You can only do your best in aiming for a natural birth, as sometimes a specific intervention is the best decision for you and your baby. However, do be ready, perhaps with your partner's help, to question decisions and ask for alternatives or options. It is reasonable to be assertive, using the knowledge you have gained during pregnancy. Be aware of your right to question any procedures you believe unnecessary.

However, you should never feel guilty or let down if you do choose or need to have a caesarean section or pain relief such as an epidural. Skin-to-skin contact and baby's climb to his first breastfeed can still be encouraged as soon as possible—especially when this has been made clear in your 'after birth feeding plan'. (Hung and Berg, 2011)

Simple suggestions to be in the best position for a natural vaginal birth are:

Health

Pay attention to your general health and eating habits. Eat healthily and avoid excessive weight gain by keeping your body fit. Regular exercise like walking and yoga are great. Attend antenatal classes if you have the opportunity—they often have specific breastfeeding sessions. Make the most of the regular doctor and midwife checks for your general well being. Be clear with your thoughts regarding your baby's birth and feeding preferences and always ask questions regarding anything that concerns you.

One of the most common complications of pregnancy that often effects baby's birth method and early feeding, is a condition called Gestational Diabetes Mellitus (GDM) It affects 5-10% of pregnant women and is related to the general rise in people being overweight. GDM develops slowly in the latter part of pregnancy and is usually detected with tests that show a mother's, and therefore her baby's higher than normal blood sugar levels. This means that both mother and baby's endocrine systems have to work much harder to make more of the hormone insulin, to manage or metabolise the sugar. One thing leads to another—babies with excess sugar put on excess weight, often becoming 30% larger, making a vaginal birth more difficult, and caesarean birth more common. Babies are more likely to be separated from mothers at birth and placed in a special care nursery, delaying the first breastfeed. Although GDM for mother is usually transitory with blood sugar levels returning to normal after baby's birth, it does have implications in future pregnancies. It also results in a higher risk of developing Diabetes Type 2. Breastfeeding reduces this risk. (Riordan and Wambach, 2010)

Note: This is a scenario where it would be particularly useful if you have expressed and saved colostrum during the last months of pregnancy as described in Chapter 2. Baby's blood sugar level will fall after birth once separated from access to your supply. He could be given your saved colostrum on a teaspoon or straight from the stored syringe—defrosted, of course. This will quickly balance his blood sugar levels and avoid him being given any other type of sustenance. Therefore, exclusive breastfeeding can be maintained.

The good thing is that GDM can be avoided or minimalised by taking extra care of your health during pregnancy. Some simple strategies are: be active every day; sit less; build strength; eat healthy meals and snacks and apply careful management of your weight gain during pregnancy.

Health care during pregnancy

When pregnant, consider your available health care system. Look at your options. Choose, if you can, one that involves people who are committed to helping you learn about the birth process. Respect for your cultural beliefs and preferences is essential, as is information that you, your partner and support people can understand and feel comfortable with. The best decisions for you and your baby can be made when you trust and communicate well with your caregivers.

Consider a *BFHI* hospital

BFHI stands for *Baby Friendly Health Initiative*. For a hospital to be accredited as *BFHI*, all staff are trained in *The Ten Steps to Successful Breastfeeding,* which aim to protect, promote and support breastfeeding (WHO, UNICEF, 2017). The number of *BFHI* hospitals in the world is increasing.

Wherever you live in the world, if you intend having your baby in a hospital and need to *book in*, you can ask whether there is a *BFHI* or a *Baby Friendly Hospital* in your area. You may be more likely to be encouraged and supported to have a natural birth, with quiet time afterwards for baby to initiate breastfeeding.

Doulas

This is a greek word meaning *woman who serves*. Doulas are good resource people during labour and birth. One-on-one support often results in higher parent satisfaction and a significant reduction in caesarean deliveries.

A doula may:

- suggest strategies for pain relief

- help partners provide useful support

- help you find comfortable positions

- explain what is happening during labour

- answer questions about the labour process

- provide tips on how to decrease stress

- assist with breastfeeding

Home birth

Non-hospital birth rates with independent midwives assisting, are rising in some countries. These are ideal for healthy women with normal uncomplicated pregnancies. If planning a home birth, it is wise to discuss with midwives what follow-up support is routinely in place or would be available if needed.

In reality, as already mentioned, there are elements of unknown about every baby's arrival. However, no matter how or where your baby is born, you can adapt aspects of your after birth feeding plan to fit your situation. Having skin-to-skin contact as soon as possible and encouraging the first significant breastfeeds are priorities.

Summary

Learning as much as you can gives a huge advantage to making informed decisions about what you and your partner would like to happen both during the birth and the immediate time after. There is less confusion when you've already decided what is best for you. More of the control is in your hands. Knowledge about the advantages of natural birth and having an *after birth feeding plan* gives you more confidence in expressing your desires, regardless of the way baby is born. Also valuable is the awareness of the advantages of baby gathering your healthy microbiome either directly, or indirectly, as after a caesarean delivery. You will also take into account the need to be realistic and flexible, as there are many different birth scenarios. It is important that medical intervention is used wisely for the best outcomes for babies and their mothers.

Chapter 4

The miraculous magical hours
How baby can crawl to his first feed

The benefits to the mother of immediate breastfeeding are innumerable, not the least of which after the weariness of labour and birth is the emotional gratification, the feeling of strength, the composure, and the sense of fulfilment that comes with the handling and suckling of the baby.—Ashley Montagu *Touching: The Human Significance of the Skin*, Second Edition, 1979

I have heard the baby's first hour after birth being referred to as the magical hour, the golden hour, or even the sacred hour. As these names suggest this is a significant time for both mother and baby.

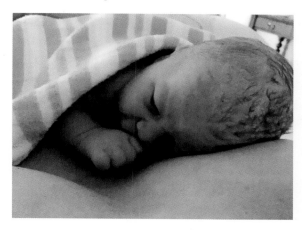

It is about you and your baby using natural instincts to connect, bond and breastfeed for the first time. It is about your partner's initial contact; the beginning of his or her close relationship. This chapter explains how the immediate time after baby's birth can be particularly beneficial.

When baby is born and is immediately placed against your bare skin, his natural reflexes and senses of hearing, sight, smell, touch and taste are elevated. During this skin-to-skin time, a fantastic series of events and movements have been observed time and time again. If left undisturbed you can watch in wonder as he wriggles or climbs (newborn *step reflex*) up your body to choose one or other of your breasts to self-attach and suckle (newborn *suck reflex*) for the very first time. Your baby knows just what to do. Sometimes this is described as the *breast crawl*. It is a beautiful and calming reward for you both after the rigorous work of labour.

This unique window of time for the 'breast crawl' is often overlooked in busy hospitals and other birthing situations, and so the 'magical hour' when that first instinctive breastfeed with baby's senses heightened is missed.

This time can be an important foundation for breastfeeding. It is as if baby's brain is programmed for effective attachment to suckle correctly. When he latches and suckles for this first time his reward will be just a few drops of colostrum. This is all he needs.

Because of its excellent value in getting breastfeeding off to a great start and because it can be a highlight of early parenting, I will describe the baby's *breast crawl* in detail. Being aware of baby's natural instincts means you can relax and observe as your new baby gradually progresses to your breast area. Watch him choose one or the other breast, before latching and suckling. This commonly happens in nine stages, and usually takes about one hour.

These stages are based on the work of international experts Ann-Marie Widstom and Lars-Ake Hanson who have produced a video of *The Magical Hour*.

- The birth cry
- Relaxation
- Awakening
- Increase in activity
- Rest
- Crawling
- Familiarisation
- Suckling
- Sleeping

The following photographs are contributions from some of the parents with whom I have had the privilege to be involved.

Stage 1. The birth cry: This is most welcome so that we all know that baby's lungs have expanded for the first time, and he is

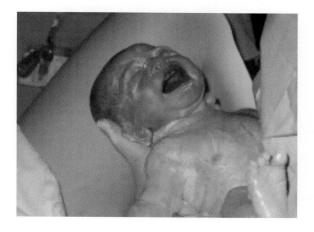

breathing. He rapidly changes colour from blueish to pink as his blood is oxygenated by the air that he is taking in. From here he is placed directly on the bare skin of your abdomen.

Stage 2. Relaxation: After his initial cry, he may have a little rest on your tummy. Possibly he is taking stock of the situation: listening, hearing your voice and heartbeat. Although familiar, they now sound different. The world outside your womb also feels very different - he is surrounded by fresh air instead of warm syrupy fluid. At this point, he doesn't move much, but his eyes may be open as he looks around. Baby can see, but his focal distance is short. He will often stare fixedly at a face. A warm towel can be placed over you both, keeping close skin-to-skin contact. Now just watch and enjoy.

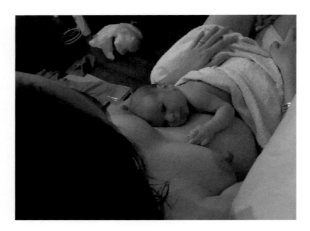

Stage 3. Awakening: Within about three minutes after birth, you may notice him move his head, shift his shoulders and wriggle his mouth. All the time, he is alert, comforted by your touch and the warmness of your skin.

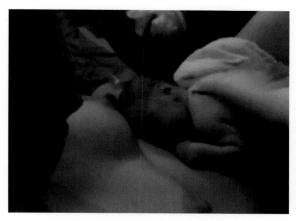

Stage 4. Increase in activity: About eight minutes after birth you may notice his body, legs and arms move more.

Stage 5. Rest: At any point during this time, baby may rest quietly, almost as if he is assessing the situation before moving on.

Stage 6. Crawling: He uses his *stepping reflex* to further move up your body. His mouth's *seeking reflex* becomes more evident as he moves his head from side to side. Your enticing mother scent may stimulate him to produce more saliva.

Approximately 35 minutes after birth, baby approaches your breast with short bursts of activity. He uses his natural instincts and reflexes as well as his heightened senses of sight, smell and touch to lead him to your breast. He may lift his head and bob around, eyes wide open, to find it. Your nipples and surrounding areas (areola) will have become darkened during the latter part of pregnancy to help with this task.

Baby's sight at birth is around seventeen centimetres. He can turn towards the light and is attracted to round features, such

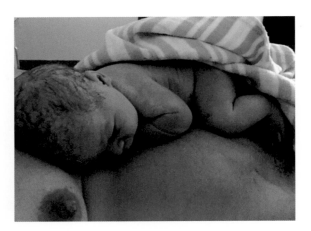

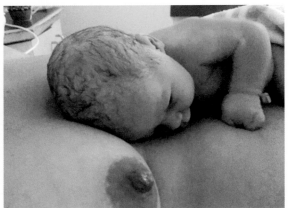

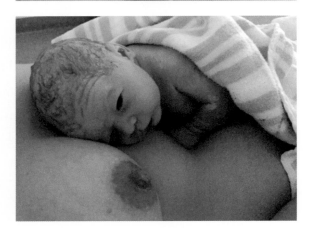

as parents' faces and the darkened area of the breast's areola and nipple. (Chilton, 2013)

Stage 7. Familiarisation: Once close to your nipple he becomes more acquainted with the area, producing more saliva, licking your nipple and his fists. This familiarisation usually begins about 45 minutes after birth and could last for 20 minutes or more. Hands are important, and he may use them to gently massage your breast. This incidentally, helps the natural passage of your placenta or afterbirth.

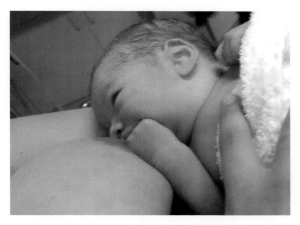

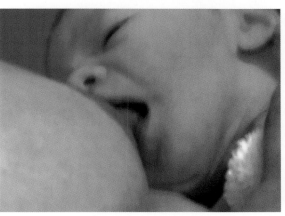

Stage 8. Suckling: Usually, within one hour after birth, baby will self-attach to one or other of your nipples and start suckling for the first time. When he self-attaches like this, it is natural for him to have his mouth and tongue in the correct position.

Breasts and nipples come in all shapes and sizes—large, small and in-between, but at this early stage, because only small amounts of colostrum are produced, they are soft and pliable for baby to attach and suckle. Because he is using his heightened instincts and newborn reflexes, he will most probably latch correctly, laying the foundation for subsequent breastfeeds. This early practice helps the long-term outlook for you both on your breastfeeding journey. If your baby has had medication transferred from you during labour as would be the case with epidural or pain drugs, he naturally may take longer to move through these stages and begin suckling. Knowing this may help you to express your desire for more quiet time to give your baby the opportunity to progress through these fascinating steps.

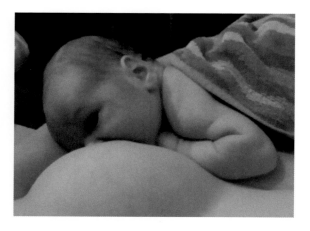

Stage 9. Sleeping: The final stage is for you to both have a restful sleep, which usually happens within about two hours after birth if left undisturbed.

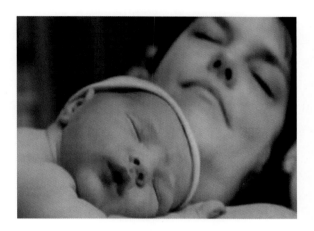

Throughout this incredible sequence of natural events, your baby is feeling warm, secure, and safe after his passage through your birth canal. He has gathered beneficial bacteria during the process to help to build his immune system and aid digestion. He can hear your heartbeat as well as your voice, feel your touch and smell your unique smell. And he is rewarded by his initial *outside drink*—a few drops of first milk or colostrum. He is on his way! This unique time after birth is described in detail because of its value in getting breastfeeding off to a positive start.

During early childhood development, there are specific windows of opportunity that, if used correctly can have far-reaching effects. The first hours after birth are such a time.

Sadly, for all sorts of reasons this knowledge is widely disregarded, possibly due to hospital 'busy-ness', lack of

Sometimes, this quiet time after birth is not possible. Or, you may try all the above suggestions, and your baby still seems uninterested in feeding. Do not, however, underestimate the foundation benefits of having quiet skin-to-skin time. It will stand you in good stead for when the baby does show interest in feeding. Do what you can, when you can. If attempted later, skin-to-skin contact (touch) is an excellent enhancer to your baby's natural instincts of sight, hearing, smell and taste, even though senses may not be as heightened as in the first hours after birth.

Babies born by caesarean

If your baby is born by caesarean section, your *after birth feeding plan* can be adapted. Ideally, you and your partner have discussed what you would like to happen with doctors and midwives. Then your partner can be an excellent advocate for you. A caesarean is considered a major operation, and consequently, more staff involvement is often needed to aid recovery and initiate breastfeeding. Many hospitals, particularly those that are BFHI accredited have breastfeeding protocols in place after caesarean operations. These can vary from hospital to hospital and according to whether you have a general anaesthetic or epidural anaesthesia for the birth. Mostly, this involves skin-to-skin contact as soon as possible, which may be in theatre or a recovery ward, where you and baby can be supported to have the first breastfeed. If this is not feasible, baby can be placed against your partner's bare chest until you have recovered sufficiently to hold him yourself.

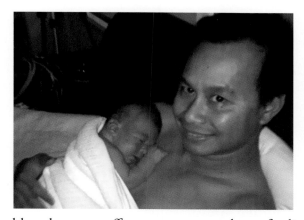

Staff should make every effort to encourage breastfeeding within the first two hours after birth and keep you and baby together unless necessary to separate you. If you are unable to sit due to pain, discomfort or nausea, midwives can help by assisting you to feed in a lying down position. If your baby has not fed in the first few hours, midwives can help you to express colostrum, which can be given to baby via a cup or spoon, thus avoiding the use of rubber teats in baby's mouth. Expressing colostrum in these particular situations is important, as it encourages the production of breastmilk.

Babies born prematurely

It is not as easy to adapt your *after birth feeding plan* if baby is born well before his due date. There are challenges that parents and babies face depending on how premature baby is. Usually, there is a far higher degree of reliance upon the specialised skills of medical and midwifery staff to guide you through this time.

Your breastmilk is of great importance to a premature baby

because it is designed to match precisely what your baby needs for the stage he is at. Your preterm milk changes according to your baby's growth. It has higher levels of protein, sodium, nitrogen, magnesium and iron, as well as increased concentrations of antimicrobial agents and immunological factors to reduce the chance of infection. It is perfect for baby's kidneys, gut, and immature brain.

The critical message for parents of premature babies is this: although daunting, breastfeeding is definitely possible and with appropriate care, even very premature babies do well. The highly skilled staff caring for you and your baby will guide you through the steps needed to initiate breastfeeding wherever possible. A significant part of this is supporting you to express your colostrum, starting as early as possible after baby's birth, with an explanation as to how breastfeeding can progress gradually. Despite the expert help, this may not be easy because of all your feelings and emotions connected with having your baby earlier than expected. However, having information about colostrum, breastmilk and knowing about breastfeeding in general, will enable you to give your baby this best possible start.

Sometimes baby can go straight to your breast, but this does depend on his size, the degree of prematurity and physical condition. Each baby is different. His *after birth feeding plan* can be used according to his specific situation. That may include a tiny tube feeding directly into his stomach or small intestine until he is a little older. Again, as in the *after birth feeding plan*, you can, wherever possible, have baby held against your chest (skin-to-skin). This is often referred to as *kangaroo care*. Depending on his particular circumstances and providing he is mature enough, you and your baby will benefit from this contact. Staff generally know the value of this close contact with parents' warmth and smell and will guide you as to how and when to do this safely.

As baby matures and progresses, your feeding plans will change. Mothers can become proficient at expressing their milk, often producing more than their baby actually needs. Starting expressing as soon as possible after baby is born is important. It helps to establish your necessary milk supply as baby transitions from tube or another feeding method, to feeding straight from the breast.

Summary

All of this is useful information to have *up your sleeve* before baby is born, as it will help you to be comfortably assertive in communicating your needs. If by chance you do have a caesarean section or baby is born earlier than expected, you know that you can adapt your *after birth feeding plan* accordingly. Most importantly, you and your partner are aware of the value of skin-to-skin contact after birth and the great enhancer of touch to encourage baby's natural instincts to self-attach for the first breastfeeds.

Chapter 5

The first few days—10 tricks of the trade

A newborn baby has only three demands. They are warmth in the arms of its mother, food from her breasts, and security in the knowledge of her presence. Breastfeeding satisfies all three.— Grantley Dick-Read

Having a brand-new baby, whether it's your first, second, third or subsequent, is always very special—they are all uniquely different. Different also are the places you spend your first days. These depend on the baby's birth situation and birthing facility. Most babies are born in hospitals and discharged within a day or two. Home birthing in many countries is becoming more popular, with a midwife following up as necessary. Regardless, the time you have with professional support is usually brief. This chapter concentrates on aspects that are helpful to know about. The aim is to make the very early days easier and enjoyable.

1. Use the time you have help wisely—ask questions

Whether in a hospital or at home, the first few days can be an invaluable time to rest and learn. Typically, midwives will assist with the new steps you take with your baby, breastfeeding being a major one. Knowledge gained during your pregnancy will give you confidence when asking questions and evaluating what feels right for you and baby. Advice may seem confusing but will be less so when you are informed and confident. It is a good idea to make it clear that you do not want your baby to have formula and that you want to breastfeed only, or *exclusively breastfeed*. Midwives and hospital staff are becoming more informed about breastfeeding encouragement and have guidelines and protocols to follow. Regardless, don't leave it to chance—state your wishes clearly.

2. Position, position, position

Although in time, most mothers work out their own particular way of holding and feeding their baby, it is useful to outline ideas that can assist you to feel more relaxed in the very beginning. Awkward positioning and incorrect attachment lead to sore nipples, discomfort and unpleasant breastfeeding. Parents are then more prone to feel tired and stressed. Correct attachment for nurturing baby is vital in helping to avoid many of the common breastfeeding obstacles discussed in Chapter 7. It is worth getting every bit of advice you can from midwives and other helpers, to establish that your baby's attachment is correct, your positioning is comfortable and that baby is feeding effectively.

There are many ways to hold and feed babies—sitting up, lying down, the *football hold* and more. And there is no definite right or wrong way, as long as you feel natural and baby is feeding well. As already mentioned, mothers over time develop their effective ways of positioning and feeding, without giving it a second thought. In the beginning, however, when you and baby are learning about breastfeeding, you may find these three methods useful: *laid-back*, *cradle hold* and *football hold* breastfeeding positions - the most commonly used in the first weeks.

Expectant mothers who looked forward to holding and feeding their baby, may have practiced with a doll or teddy following these guidelines.

Laid-back breastfeeding

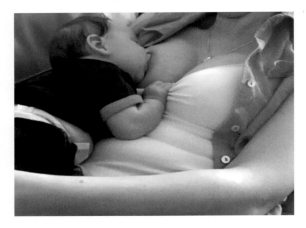

Firstly, remember your first feed after your baby was born? You were lying back a little with your new baby against your chest, skin-to-skin. This positioning is called *laid-back breastfeeding*, or *biological nurturing*. It is an ideal way to continue feeding if you choose, as long as you are comfortable, with your head and shoulders well supported. This position encourages baby to use his natural feeding reflexes. It is also handy if you have had a caesarean birth as baby can lie diagonally across your body away from your wound, while still being supported by your arm and hands around his torso and feet.

By placing baby against your front with his nose facing your nipple and his legs flexed comfortably, gravity will help him mould himself against your body He can use his hands and feet to stabilise himself. His hands help him find and shape the breast, stimulating milk to flow. As he opens his mouth wide to attach, bring him firmly inwards with your hand supporting his back, rather than his head. His chin comes into your breast more, giving him access to a good mouthful of breast to start suckling. His nose just touches your breast.

Cradle hold

Many mothers start breastfeeding by cuddling baby in their arms in a *cradle hold*. To feed in this position, pay attention to your posture— wriggle to get as comfortable as you can—even sit upright with your back supported if this feels right for you. You can have your feet firmly on the floor or stool, making your lap flat.

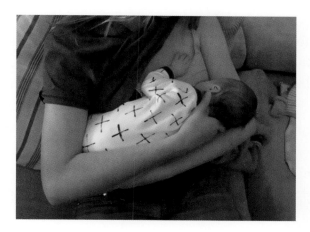

Undress baby (and yourself) as much as the temperature allows so that you and your baby have plenty of skin-to-skin contact when feeding. Again, this helps with his natural feeding instincts. Positioning baby longways across your body with his chest facing you, hold him in close with your forearm, and your hand spread widely at the top of his shoulders (not his head). This allows his head to extend back a little. With his head extended like this, his tongue will move forward over his lower gums, where it needs to be for latching to feed.

> *Just as we need to extend our heads upwards when we thirstily drink a glass of water, so it is for babies when they feed. You can experiment with this by drinking a glass of water with your head down. Notice how your tongue draws back instead of forward. It feels awkward and uncomfortable.*

Have your nipple pointing to his top lip, or even his nose. To encourage him to open his mouth widely, tease his bottom lip with the adjacent part of the areola. As he opens his mouth widely, bring him into your breast firmly, using your forearm along the back of his body and your hand at the top of his shoulders, (not head). In this position his chin and bottom lip will meet the breast first, three to four centimetres below or to the central side of your nipple (depending on the exact cradle hold positioning). His tongue will be over his lower gums. This way he can draw a large part of the areola, as well as the nipple into his mouth. The nipple, being quite elastic, ends up towards the back of baby's mouth where his soft palate starts. When this happens, no damage to your nipple can occur, and feeding is efficient and comfortable.

> *Again, experiment by feeling your own soft palate with your tongue or finger. When your nipple is in this position in baby's mouth, his tongue can easily remove your milk or colostrum with a rhythmic rolling front to back action. All the necessary face and jaw muscles needed for breastfeeding are being used.*

Attachment—The key to successful Breastfeeding

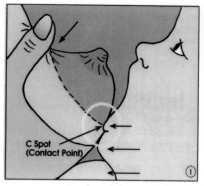
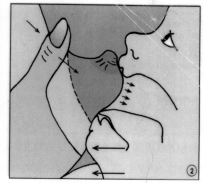

Firmly push between baby's shoulders, bringing baby onto the breast

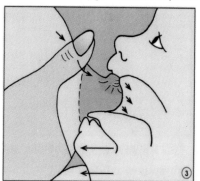
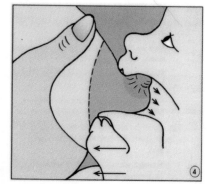

The breast completely fills baby's mouth

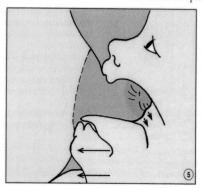
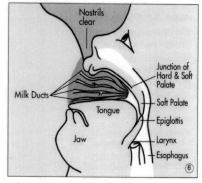

This triggers baby's suckling reflexes

The above diagrams are from Western Australian Lactation Consultant Rebecca Glover's *The Key to Successful Breastfeeding* pamphlet and are used with her permission, to clearly illustrate baby's attachment.

Note that many women say that in the first week, even if baby is attaching correctly, there is a degree of nipple discomfort as breasts get used to their new task. Be assured however, that it is not for long and is usually eased by spreading a little colostrum or milk around your nipples at the end of each feed. Letting your breasts air-dry before covering also helps.

Football hold

Many mothers find this comfortable, especially after a caesarean section as the wound area can be easily avoided.

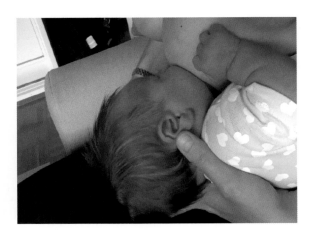

Have baby lying at your side, facing you, with his feet towards your back — a pillow may be useful to support his body, but the majority of support is from your forearm along the back of his body with your hand spread widely at the top of his shoulders. Bring him close, teasing or just touching his bottom lip on your nipple and areola area which will cause him to open his mouth widely. At that moment, use your arm to bring him firmly to your breast, chin and bottom lip first, allowing him to take in a mouthful of areola and nipple.

3. What does the correct attachment look like?

You will quickly get to know when your baby is attached and feeding well—it will be pain-free and comfortable. The actual appearance of baby feeding will be a little different according to your positioning, but generally, you will see that his whole face—

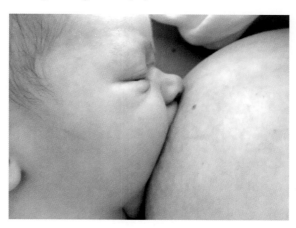

chin, cheeks, mouth and nose are close into your breast (as in the photographs). His chin especially is well into your breast, sometimes giving the appearance of him having a *double chin* as he feeds. His nose is touching, or just off the breast, and his head is tilted slightly upward from his body. You might see slight movement at the base of his ears as he suckles. You may be able to observe lips widely flanged as in the following photo, but more often lips will be well-embedded in the close contact of breast tissue. The mother/baby *fit* when breastfeeding can be different for everyone because of the diversity of breast and nipple shapes and sizes, and aspects of baby's mouth and chin. Mostly, it is evident that baby's attachment is correct simply when it *feels right* and you can hear baby swallowing, particularly in the first part of his feed.

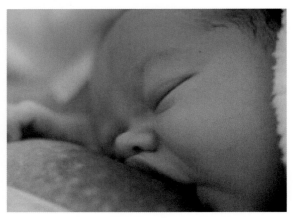

4. Colostrum—How much does he need?

If your hospital time is short (two days or less), babies suckle only small amounts of colostrum. Their tiny stomachs only hold half a teaspoon in the first feed and one or two teaspoons in subsequent feeds. This small amount is all he needs. Sometimes parents worry that this is not enough for their baby. It is reassuring to know that he has extra body tissue fluids and pads of *brown fat* around his shoulders and neck. Baby uses these fluids and fat to provide additional nourishment while he makes the transition from being fed in your womb to being fed breastmilk via your breasts.

The diagrams below from Ameda Belly Balls Lactation Tool (Nancy Mohrbacher, 2002) will help you visualise just how big baby's stomach is at birth, which reinforces the fact that small frequent breastfeeds of colostrum are more than enough to meet baby's needs. These balls have been used for many years by midwives to demonstrate the size of babies' stomachs at birth.

Shooter Marble	=	Approximate stomach capacity of a newborn on Day 1
Ping Pong Ball	=	Approximate stomach capacity on Day 3
Extra-Large Chicken Egg	=	Approximate stomach capacity on Day 10
Softball	=	Approximate stomach capacity of an adult

Shooter Marble 5-7 ml

Ping Pong Ball 22-27 ml

Extra-Large Chicken Egg 60-81 ml

Babies are born with quite immature immune systems and depend on colostrum to coat the lining of their digestive tract with high concentrations of nutrients and antibodies. It is nourishing and prevents bacteria crossing into his blood, inhibiting infection. Colostrum also stimulates the movement in baby's bowel (peristalsis) to pass his first 'poo'. This first bowel action is black and sticky and is called *meconium*.

5. Colostrum to milk—what to expect.

By the second, third or fourth day, colostrum transitions to more mature milk. Baby's stomach capacity gradually increases with frequent small feedings until by day ten it holds approximately 60 to 80 mls.

As this happens, you will notice your baby's bowel actions change. His first bowel action is that sticky black *meconium*, but this changes over the next few days to a greeny-black colour, then to a greeny-brown and eventually to a mustard-yellow colour by about the fourth or fifth day.

You will also notice your breasts changing. They will become fuller until, by the second or third day, you will be in the transition stage of your breastmilk production. Sometimes we hear stories about *when the milk comes in* with breasts being *engorged and painful*. At this time your breasts do become more distended due to tissue fluid and an increased blood supply needed for making milk. Sometimes the tissue fluid is excessive due to intravenous fluids that you may have had during the birthing process.

Discomfort caused by filling and full breasts can be reduced enormously by encouraging baby to feed frequently. The more often he feeds, the less discomfort occurs, especially in the first few days. Of course, proper attachment to the breast is a huge help. This is why the first breastfeed soon after birth that can *program* baby's brain for the correct way to latch is so useful. Babies usually lose a small amount of weight as they transition from colostrum to the more mature breastmilk. This is normal and should not be interpreted as needing anything extra in the way of nutrition.

It is important to know that some initial weight loss is normal. Sometimes it can be misinterpreted, leading to baby being given formula from a bottle, which should only be necessary under exceptional circumstances. It can lead to undesirable changes in baby's gut bacteria and confusion between sucking on the teat of a bottle and suckling at the breast.

6. How often to feed?

A rough guide to aim for are between eight and twelve breastfeeds in 24 hours, so that is about two hourly. Not all babies show a keen interest in feeding in the early days. They are all different. Feeds can be encouraged with cuddling skin-to-skin, close to your breast where your smell and touch enhance the natural feeding instincts. Frequent feeds are beneficial to you as you learn about your baby, and your baby learns about you. By feeding baby frequently you are reinforcing attaching techniques and your breasts get a clear message to transition from colostrum to mature milk.

In the first days and weeks, feed as often as you think your baby wants, without restriction or timing. Watch him for signs or *cues* that he is ready to feed, making it *baby-led*, not *clock-led*. Signs include moving his arms and body more, perhaps hands towards his mouth or subtle lip movements.

7. Just breast

In these early days and weeks, there is no need for anything to go into your baby's mouth except breast and breastmilk: no water, no formula, no rubber teats and no dummies. Sucking on artificial teats is very different from suckling on your breast. Sucking on the teat requires almost no effort—he uses fewer facial muscles and different tongue positioning than he does when breastfeeding. When baby goes to the breast after having sucked on a dummy or the teat of a bottle, he can become confused and treat your nipple like the dummy, squashing it up against the hard roof of his mouth. This can lead to pain and discomfort, as your nipples are very sensitive. Sore nipples, along with a baby who is confused or fussy with breastfeeding, may make you doubt your ability to breastfeed. *Breast only* will mean that your baby can build on what he learned in the first breastfeeds after birth. With just breastmilk, he will quickly grow strong facial and jaw muscles to enable him to feed in the beautiful way nature intended.

After breastfeeding is established, (which generally takes approximately six weeks), provided your baby is gaining weight, and you are comfortable feeding, dummies or pacifiers should not cause any confusion. Baby's face and jaw muscles needed for breastfeeding will be well developed, and he should not be 'confused' by switching between breast and dummy.

8. Involving partners

It can be genuinely daunting for partners as they participate and support you through labour and birth. Ideally, you are a tight team, and the experience is a highlight for both of you. After baby's birth, the focus is usually on mother, baby and feeding, feeding, feeding. So for a partner, the reality may be very different from imagined. There may be feelings of being *left out* or excluded. Partners or fathers play such an important role in breastfeeding success because of the support they can give. It is invaluable. Encouragement for partners to participate will increase their confidence, and enable them to give appreciative and positive feedback. The connection or bond between partner and baby will grow more quickly when you are both involved, leading to parental closeness and better breastfeeding outcomes.

> *As Alyssa Schnell says about partners in her book,* Breastfeeding Without Birthing:-*Your support of breastfeeding is a life-long gift you can give your baby and your partner. It only seems like breastfeeding is a one-person job!*

9. Understanding the *Third Day Blues*

About day three to five after baby's birth, many women will notice a sudden drop in mood, often for no apparent reason. This can be distressing for a mother, her partner and caregivers. Feelings of anxiety, sadness or being overwhelmed can seem strange after the elation of the baby's birth. It is useful to know that these feelings are common and usually pass quickly. Considering the tremendous hormonal changes that occur, all in a short space of days, these mood changes are understandable. Significant body adjustments happen as hormones needed for pregnancy exit your body just as others are being *turned on* to start your milk production. Knowing that they peak at about one week then taper off by the end of the second week can be reassuring and lessen their impact. If these feelings persist for more than two weeks after baby's birth, it is worth speaking to someone you trust, perhaps someone on your *resource list.*

If negative feelings do not subside, there is more chance of them developing into the more challenging condition of Post Natal Depression (Smith, 2018). *This is discussed further in Chapter 7.*

10. Confidence

Mothers need support as focus shifts away from the labour and birth to the new baby. The reality is that it is not always easy to *bounce back* quickly. Ideally, the time after baby's birth is for slowing down and being nurtured, with a balance of eating, drinking, resting and feeding. Too many visitors can be exhausting.

Even the most experienced and competent person can be surprised at how confidence can waver. The changes that childbirth brings can be overwhelming. Interrupted sleep, hormones that are trying to settle into a pattern, other siblings and all the other demands in life, can make it hard to stay *on top of the world* all the time. Not to mention the confusing, but well-meant advice that can come your way! You may think, It's just you who is faltering—this is not the case. Remember, you don't have to be *on top of the world* all the time. It is quite normal to feel the highs and lows as you, your baby and family settle into any new situation.

Again, partners can play a large part in boosting confidence. Partners can let new mothers know what a brilliant job they are doing. The small things can make such a difference. A comforting hug can give a boost. Keeping loads of visitors away, staying ahead of household chores, or ensuring a drink is handy when baby is feeding, are useful ideas. When partners can nurture the new mother, as well as look after their own health and well-being, confidence grows.

Additionally, the sharing of parenting can become more relaxed and enjoyable.

In all of this, I am assuming there are two parents involved. This is not necessarily the case as many will choose, or be in a situation, to parent alone. There are so many different parenting scenarios that are equally important and special. Parenting challenges can be different, but the outcome for mother and baby can be just as positive. Ideally, nurturing supports and resources are gathered during pregnancy and then used and appreciated as life with your baby unfolds.

11. And one for luck: use your resources

Remember when you were pregnant, planning for this baby, you wrote down a list of useful contacts? These contacts will be aligned with where you live—city or country, and what is available to you. If you wish to discuss any aspect of breastfeeding, parenting, your general health or the way you are feeling, do not hesitate to use that list. Phone or go to the people or organisations that you think will meet your needs. Nothing is insignificant or unimportant. Do not stop until you have the appropriate help and information. Chapter 13 details some of the more general useful resources.

Breastfeeding often requires explicit support—it is not always easy to find, and many mothers give up and move to formula feeding unnecessarily because they do not use, or do not know where to go for the right help. You and your baby's health and well-being are paramount. Two well-known, reliable resources are: La Leche League International[1] and The Australian Breastfeeding Association.[2]

1 www.llli.org/get-help
2 www.breastfeeding.asn.au

Summary

It's good to be aware that after your baby's birth, frequent feeding is ideal (between 8 and 12 times in 24 hours). Take care with attaching baby to feed (See the diagrams of positioning). A small amount of colostrum in the first few days is all he needs, as he has a tiny tummy. Avoid additional supplementation unless medically indicated as it can be detrimental to breastfeeding outcomes. Be aware that you may feel a drop in mood on about day three, and that this is normal and should resolve. Talk, discuss, involve your partner as much as possible. Do not be confused by well-meant advice from friends, relatives or acquaintances—let it go in one ear and out the other as you nod and say, *thank you*. Don't hesitate to seek advice from those on your *resource list* to clarify any queries you may have. Most of all, enjoy this somewhat fleeting time of beautiful beginnings with your new baby.

Chapter 6

The first few weeks—useful knowledge

Breastfeeding is an instinctual and natural act, but it is also an art that is learned day by day. The reality is that almost all women can breastfeed, have enough milk for their babies and learn how to overcome problems both large and small. It is almost always simply a matter of practical knowledge and not a question of good luck.—La Leche League

The birth is over—your baby is born. What you have been anticipating with extreme interest and perhaps anxiety is now behind you, and you are on to the next big part—recalibrating yourself mentally and physically and settling into life with your new baby and new family dynamics. You have probably been with midwives or other caring people who have answered questions and given you information, support and encouragement. You may be back in the comfort and familiarity of your own home and may or may not have help in the way of a supportive partner. Regardless, the first few weeks can be daunting, particularly if it is your first baby. There seems so much to think about, and the responsibility can feel overwhelming. This chapter is about continuing to build on a good foundation and unravelling the most common queries in the first weeks.

This is often the time when women lose confidence in their ability to breastfeed and question whether what they are doing is correct, or 'normal'. So it is a critical time to use the knowledge gained during pregnancy to put things into perspective calmly. If in any doubt, or if niggling concerns become worries do not hesitate to contact a trusted person.

All mother and baby pairs are different and unique and what is happening for one mother, will be different for another. However, these are the most common questions that my colleagues and I have been asked by new parents as they settle into life with their new baby.

How often should I be feeding?

Breastfeeding takes much of your time and energy in the early weeks. This is normal. At times it may feel that as soon as one feed finishes, it's almost time to start another. This may be tiring at first, but it does give you and your baby opportunity to practice how it all works. It also gives your breasts a firm message that they are very much needed to do what nature intended. Breastmilk digests very quickly, so frequent feeding is necessary to satisfy not only hunger but also the need to feel warm, close and secure with you. So again, follow your baby, not the clock. Each time you feed, see it as a restful time-out for you and your baby.

It does help if you create a 'feeding station', or a spot in your home where you can be particularly comfortable with everything you need nearby. For example, phone, drink, something to read, somewhere to put your feet up. If there are older siblings, a bag or box of special toys that come out at feeding time can be handy.

Usually in the first weeks baby will feed as often as two to three hourly, night and day. This does vary from mother to mother as milk storage capacity in her breasts can play a part in how often a baby feeds. Some breasts hold larger amounts of milk and babies quickly get used to having bigger meals, and so may not need to feed as often. Other breasts hold smaller amounts, so babies need to have more frequent but smaller feed amounts. It doesn't matter what size your breasts are, or how much they hold. There is always an adequate supply of milk that will be taken at different time intervals if you follow your baby's hungry signs or cues.

Feeding cues vary from baby to baby. Usually, each mother learns her baby's particular, sometimes subtle, signs. It is a good idea to pick baby up to cuddle and feed before feeding cues become too obvious. Crying is a late feeding sign. Babies feed better if they are offered a feed before they get to the crying stage. Early signs that baby is ready for a feed are likely to be fidgeting or squirming, stretching, turning head, opening the mouth, putting a hand towards or in the mouth, or generally fussing.

Every mother and baby will eventually develop their own feeding pattern. Often it changes from day to day and week to week, as baby grows. There is a huge variation in what is *normal*. It is a great asset to you and your baby to be as relaxed as possible about how often your baby feeds. In fact, some parents don't even think about *how often*, they just follow their baby's hungry signs or needs, which usually become clearer as time passes.

Because breastmilk is such perfectly balanced nutritionally, it is easily digested. Breastmilk leaves baby's stomach empty after about thirty-five minutes (Chilton, 2017). *This is one of the reasons babies need to feed frequently—even hourly at times. They don't 'watch the clock', they only respond to their feelings, which may be hunger, but could also be a need to feel your warm, comfortable closeness; to feel secure. A breastfeed fulfils all these needs. It may be a short feed or a more lengthy affair, but trust your baby to be the leader in this—he knows his needs. As time passes, as already mentioned, breastfeeding becomes quicker and easier. Each time it is an opportunity for you to relax and rest.*

Night feeds

Over the first weeks and months, parents often become quite tired from all the changes in their lives and the interrupted sleep. They may yearn for a good night's sleep and ask the question—When will my baby sleep through the night? Importantly you need to know that it is very normal for a baby to wake during the night for feeds. It is also good to know that the sometimes frequent night feeds that occur in the early weeks do not continue forever! Generally, babies get the gist of day and night after a few weeks, and night feeds become more spaced giving you longer stretches of sleep. If this does not occur naturally, babies can be encouraged to get their day and night *sorted*, as explained below.

More sleep at night?

Somewhere in a twenty-four hour period, most babies will have one longer stretch of sleep time. This may be a four, five or even six-hour stretch of sleep. If babies happen to have this longer sleep during the day, they probably won't have it at night, which means they will wake for more frequent night feeds. If this becomes a regular occurrence and baby is waking, for example, every two or three hourly for a feed during the night and having a longer stretch of sleep sometime during the day, you may wish to encourage a change in his pattern.

You can do this by cutting short that longer day sleep. After about three hours from his last feed, gently wake by picking him up for a cuddle and a *talk*. You will usually find that fairly quickly he will let you know that he is ready for a breastfeed by bringing his hands to his mouth, moving his head from side to side or perhaps starting to *grizzle*. In this way, you can encourage a pattern of feeding more frequently in the day than during the night. Helping baby get his day/night pattern sorted by ensuring he is feeding reasonably often during the day will encourage that longer stretch of sleep at night.

We all need our sleep, and because night feeds are part of the whole new baby package, it means that you need to use all of the *tricks of the trade* to make feeding at night as easy as possible for you, your baby and your partner. Having baby's cot in your room (room sharing) is an ideal way to have baby close. You can feed, and return him to his cot for sleep when finished, with minimal disruption. When mother and baby are close they will often develop a similar sleep rhythm and stir from sleep at the same time.

As well as meeting baby's needs for comfort and nourishment, night feeds most probably delay your menstrual cycle, due to the natural suppression of the hormones that stimulate ovulation. Feeds during the night have a contraceptive effect. Providing baby is under six months of age, is exclusively breastfed, is feeding reasonably often during the day and has one or two night feeds, ovulation and therefore menstruation is unlikely to occur. (Mohrbacher, 2012) *Regardless, it is good to be aware that every woman is different, so other means of contraception may be required.*

To wrap, or not to wrap?

In the early days of feeding, you may find baby's arms are going everywhere. They seem to hinder or get in the way of attaching properly to feed. Admittedly when you are both learning about breastfeeding, it is frustrating when baby seems to want to suck hands, as well as attach and feed. In the past, it has been very common to swaddle baby with hands tucked well away, but recent research (Genna and Barak, 2015) has questioned this practice for several reasons. It is thought that baby's hands for them are like a tool to help steady or stabilise themselves against the breast. Before attaching to feed, they may pummel or push at the breast. This encourages the hormone oxytocin to increase, causing nipples to become more erect. Baby's hands can move and shape the breast, making it easier to attach. Sometimes they seem to circle or wave around until they settle against your skin. Baby may use his hands to push back away from your breast so that he can get a better view of the nipple and areolar area. He may even feel your nipple with his hand and then use it as a guide to bring him in closer to attach and feed. As breastfeeding progresses, baby's arms and hands have more control; they go to the breast area but do not get in the way of attaching to feed.

It may be helpful, rather than wrapping arms and hands away, to have assistance to gently move baby's hand slightly, until he is attached properly to feed. He will quickly learn where to place his hands for feeding efficiency. Wrapping, or swaddling can be a useful strategy to help baby settle for sleeps, as described fully in Chapter 10.

One breast or two?

Whether to use one breast or two is a common query. In the very early days with babies' stomachs being so small, they are often satisfied and sleepy after feeding on one breast. As the days go by, however, and your milk supply increases, baby's stomach size and appetite also increase. It is, therefore, a good idea to always offer the baby the second side at each feed time—or ensure baby starts on that second side for the next feed. Each side should get regular stimulation and emptying. Remember every mother/baby couple is different and there is a wide variation in what is *normal*. One mother may go through her whole lactation period happily feeding on one breast per feed. However, most babies will take from both sides every feed.

A strategy that often works is to change baby's nappy or have a short cuddle between sides. Breastmilk digests quickly. A brief break allows time for milk from the first breast to 'move along', making it more likely that he will be keen to have more from the second breast.

Is my baby getting enough?

As time goes on, you may be surprised at how very quick breastfeeds become—at how super efficient your baby is at having what he needs. Initially, feeds may seem time-consuming—anything up to an hour. Although the time it takes to feed baby does vary, often feeds can become remarkedly quick. This is a time you might wonder—has he really had enough? Be reassured that he most probably has. There are many subtle ways you can tell that baby is getting all that he needs for perfect growth and development. One of the main signs is baby's behaviour at the end of feeding. If he disengages from your breast in his own time, looking relaxed, sleepy and content, it is a good sign. Babies arrive with their own inbuilt appetite control system, taking from you only what their bodies need. Babies don't overfeed on breastmilk, and the amount they have each feed can vary. Feel confident that you fed your baby for nine months perfectly in your womb, and there is no reason for this not to continue for as long as you both want.

If ever in doubt, offer him more. He will attach and suckle again if he does need more. If he takes a little more than he needs, he will likely have a little *spill* at some point. It is common for babies to regurgitate small amounts of milk. It doesn't mean that you need to feed again to replace the milk that has been *spilt*.

Another sign that he is getting enough is his output—usually six or so wet nappies in 24 hours. *Poos* can vary—some babies have a small soft yellow bowel action almost every time they feed. This is common in the very early weeks. As time passes, bowel movements become less frequent. One a day to one every few days, to even one a week is within normal limits.

Weight gain is another sign that baby is getting enough. Usually by two weeks of age, baby has regained the weight he lost after birth and is back to, or above his birth weight. So often a baby who has had a great start breastfeeding, and feeds comfortably and frequently, will surpass his birth weight very quickly. It is obvious that he is getting enough.

Baby's weight gain—What should it be?

Many parents do worry about whether their baby is gaining weight adequately. Often it is an unnecessary concern and based on comparisons with others. All babies have different genetic makeup, and their growth will vary accordingly. If healthy, as most babies are, they gain weight in a way that is right for them. Frequent weighing is not necessary. The best indicator of growth and development is how your baby looks and behaves. His feeds, sleep and general disposition are the main indications of his progress.

As a general guide babies will:

- Lose weight in the first few days but regain to their birth weight by two weeks of age; many surpass birth weight

- Double their weight by five months, triple by twelve months and quadruple it by two years

- Increase their length by 2.5cm each month in the first six months, then by 1.25cm a month in the second six months

> Be aware of the World Health Organisation WHO growth charts in your baby's health record book. They give an overall picture of progress when weight and length are charted at varying intervals. A good time to review progress and chart measurements is at the recommended health check times, which are slightly different in each country – or, of course, any other time if you are concerned.

It is a good idea to take your baby's health record book with you whenever he is getting checked. Make sure his measurements are entered and charted in his book.

Do I need to *burp* my baby?

Burping or *winding* babies is something that many parents tend to do, during and at the end of the feed time. We do not really need to do this, because *wind* or *gas* occurs when the milk mixes with gastric juices as it is digested. Not because of air taken in when baby feeds. When baby is attached and is feeding well, there is a *seal* between baby's mouth and breast, so baby only swallows milk, not air. It is interesting that in many cultures parents do not *burp* babies and they have minimal trouble with them being *windy* or unsettled. However, it must be a comforting feeling for babies when they are gently put over a shoulder and cuddled, or sat up having their back rubbed. It can quickly become an expected routine. The main point to remember is that it isn't actually necessary, so don't worry if a burp doesn't evolve with those upright cuddles. Babies generally cope well, managing burping in their own time if needed, or by passing wind between or with bowel actions.

Fluctuations in feeding frequency

Often parents will notice that there are times of the day when baby seems to need feeds closer together. Commonly this happens in the late afternoon and into the evening and can be referred to as *cluster feeding*. (Bonyata, 2017). It can be quite exhausting for mothers towards the end of long, busy days, but good to know that it is considered normal. Perhaps it is baby's way of stocking up a bit before a longer interval between feeds during the night. Again, do not think that there is anything wrong with your milk supply. Extra milk from any other source will only complicate matters. This is perhaps a time where lots of close cuddles along with the more frequent, often short, feeds is what is needed. A baby carrier for you or your partner can be particularly useful. The movement and closeness can be very settling. There are also specific times—usually over two or three days, when breastfed babies do seem more hungry around the clock. These are thought to be when baby has a growth surge. Often this is around six weeks and twelve weeks, and again, should not be considered that your milk supply is diminishing. Your milk supply fluctuates to meet this extra demand, and then gradually settles to meet the lesser demand when these growth needs are met.

My breasts don't feel as full, is this a problem?

After the initial weeks of breastfeeding, mothers will often notice that their breasts feel softer and not as full. This is quite normal and is usually a sign that milk production is established and has settled to match baby's needs. Supply might rise and fall over time, according to baby's needs, but breast fullness is not usually experienced in quite the same way as in the early weeks.

Do certain foods affect my milk?

Your baby, to a great extent, is familiar with what you normally eat as he had access to your diet for the months he was in your womb. There are many myths about what not to eat while breastfeeding. However, there is no real evidence that any particular food eaten causes problems with baby's digestion. The general rule is to eat a proper diet of fruit, vegetables, cereal, dairy products, fish, meat or vegetarian alternatives, with plenty of variety and all in moderation. It is sensible to do this anyway, for your own health and well being. You may find that if you have a large amount of any one thing, for example, chocolate, orange juice or cabbage, there may be temporary changes in baby's digestion and behaviour. The important factors are moderation, eating a well-balanced diet and not avoiding anything you usually have.

Another interesting aspect to consider is that because baby has *a taste* of whatever his mother eats through small traces in her breastmilk, it often leads to baby taking to different tastes and foods more easily when introduced to solids at around six months of age. Babies are often less fussy because they have already experienced a wide variety of flavours. Formula-fed babies are disadvantaged, as milk always tastes the same and does not reflect the mother's diet.

Drinking is also important, and the best thing to drink regularly is clean tap water. You do not need to drink any specific amount— people often think you need to drink more than usual to maintain your breastmilk supply. That is not so. Drink according to your thirst, which probably will be higher than before you had your baby. Many mothers comment that they feel particularly thirsty as they breastfeed, so it is a sensible strategy always to have a large glass of water handy as you are feeding.

What about alcohol?

As mentioned in Chapter 2, a small percentage of alcohol does freely pass into your breastmilk, but if enjoyed in extreme moderation (that is an occasional drink), it is thought not to affect the baby or your milk supply. The alcohol content in your breastmilk will peak thirty to sixty minutes after you have consumed it so you can time your feed to avoid that period. It naturally passes out of your milk in two to three hours. Once again, moderation is important. Over-consumption of alcohol can have a detrimental effect on baby's growth and development, as well as your milk supply and general health.

In the first weeks you may notice:

Milia: These are tiny white spots that appear on baby's nose and cheeks soon after birth. They are due to the initial activation of baby's sweat glands and disappear within a week or two.

Normal newborn baby rash: At about three weeks of age (and usually three weeks of beautiful skin), babies, whether breastfed or not, commonly develop a red raised rash on their faces, which can be a concern to parents. It is not related to anything that you have or have not done but is simply due to baby's withdrawal from access to your hormones that he had via your blood supply while in your womb. It seems to take about this time to manifest as this *juvenile acne*. No treatment is needed, and the rash usually goes within a week or two.

Pink stained nappies: Also relating to your hormone withdrawal, is the appearance of temporary orangy-pink or blood like stains in baby's nappy. This may be noticed in the first few days after birth. It is not blood causing the colouring, but harmless chemicals called *urates* that babies initially pass in their urine.

Baby's 'poos' and 'wees': Knowing what to expect in nappies in the first weeks and beyond can stop niggling concerns about what is *normal*. Over the first few days, providing baby is feeding well his bowel actions will change. As already mentioned, his first at, or soon after birth, will be the sticky black *meconium*. It changes to a dark green, then to a greeny-brown colour by about day three. By about day four, when breastmilk supply is increasing, you can expect to see *poos* becoming lighter in colour, eventually changing to a mustardy-yellow colour. They may appear seedy, or watery. Baby will have about four wet nappies a day. By day five as milk supply and baby's intake further increases, there will be on average three to four soft, mustard-yellow *poos* in twenty-four hours and around five wet nappies.

Jaundice

Jaundice is when some babies' eyes and skin appear slightly yellow on about the third day after birth. It is due to the normal action of baby's liver breaking down or processing surplus red blood cells that he has in his body following his time in your womb. In doing so, bilirubin is released, which colours his skin. It is often noticed in the first weeks before gradually subsiding. It generally needs no action.

Occasionally, the level of bilirubin remains high. If so, it can be measured by a simple blood test and treated if necessary. Treatment is usually phototherapy for twenty-four hours. (Baby is placed under a special lamp with his eyes covered when he is sleeping). He is also encouraged to feed as much as possible. These two actions help to flush out the bilirubin from his system, resolving jaundice quickly.

Summary

There are so many new things to notice, learn and be fascinated by in the first few weeks, as you get to know your baby. It is a time of transition. Generally, there is a steep learning curve for parents, even if it is not your first baby. Babies are all different and have their unique qualities. It is also a time of recovery from the birth and the many changes in your body. Importantly, it is a time when breastfeeding is becoming established. Fathers and other non-birth partners too are adjusting as they make new connections and manage the changes in family dynamics. Understandably, there may be a significant emotional impact on parents during this time. Knowing about these aspects can be helpful in eliminating the need to be concerned unnecessarily about anything, leaving you free to enjoy the early weeks. In reality, they pass so quickly.

Chapter 7

Don't let the common 'humps' throw you
How to avoid, manage or overcome them

It's an unusual mother who experiences no bumps on the road to happy breastfeeding. The important thing is to keep going.— Dr Howard Chilton *'Baby on Board'*

I persevered through bumps in the road, to say the least with breastfeeding, because I just felt it was such a natural, beautiful, generous, organic, animal, existential, biological imperative.— Singer-songwriter Alanis Morissette

This chapter explains the most common challenges, and how they can influence the progress of breastfeeding. One of my main reasons for writing about them is to make the point that they need not cause you to give up breastfeeding. They can always be overcome using this and other information that you have gathered, and by using whoever is appropriate on your *resource list*. If it is your first baby, successfully overcoming challenges will usually make breastfeeding easier if there is a *next time*.

Don't expect problems with breastfeeding.

Many mothers that I know breeze through their breastfeeding journeys without a hitch. They love breastfeeding their babies.

So you may never come across any of the difficulties mentioned in this chapter, especially if you have been able to have skin-to-skin contact and baby-led attachment for the first breastfeed.

From experience however, I know there will be some parents who will face challenges. The global statistics attest to this. Most women leave hospital exclusively breastfeeding (around 90 per cent), but by three months more than half have introduced formula or are formula feeding. Often this is not what parents want, and it can be extremely distressing for those who have their hearts set on breastfeeding their baby. By having some knowledge of the most common difficulties that can arise, parents are better equipped and more confident to avoid, overcome or take any action necessary.

The following are common concerns based on what I have observed over the years working with parents and babies. These are the situations that drive parents to introduce formula, putting their breastfeeding goals at risk.

Sore nipples

One of the most common complaints of breastfeeding mothers is that their nipples are sore and feeding is uncomfortable. Some women do not experience any nipple discomfort during the first days of nursing. Those that do, usually find it subsiding within the first week. Initial sore nipples may be part of nature's plan to help stimulate milk production, but persistence beyond a few days indicates something is not quite right.

If discomfort grows and nipples become painful, feeding baby will be far from enjoyable. Painful nipples are really painful! And stressful. Stress is exhausting, and it is understandable that, if pain persists, feeding via the breast will not continue for long. Feeding discomfort often leads to other problems, such as nipple deterioration, the introduction of formula and a downward spiral of feeding confidence.

Nipples do damage easily and will react if baby is not attached correctly. What you feel will give a clear message if something is not right. Messages may be...*feeding doesn't feel comfortable*, or *my nipples sting after a feed*, or they *just feel tender*, or *they are really, really painful throughout a feed*. It might be that you feel *shooting pains in your breasts after a feed*. It is useful to be able to describe the pain or discomfort so that help can match the cause. Never put up with it, thinking that it is normal. The problem is often resolved instantly with adjustment in baby's positioning and attachment.

As already mentioned, sore nipples are usually related to the way baby is feeding at the breast. Often it is because your nipples are not back far enough in baby's mouth and he consequently has a *shallow latch*. As a result, as he feeds, your nipples are rubbing against the roof of his mouth or *hard palate*, instead of the soft part at the back – the *soft palate*. If this is the case, you will notice when baby comes off your breast after feeding, that your nipple will have a pinched, cone shape (like a new lipstick), rather than its regular pre-feed shape. No wonder it hurts!

If baby had his first breastfeed in that planned, skin-to-skin *golden hour* time after birth, his brain may well be *programmed* to attach well, with feeding progressing smoothly. If baby hasn't had anything in his mouth other than breast (no pacifiers, or rubber teats), he only learns one way to suck—on the breast. These two factors stand him in good stead, and sore nipples are not usually a problem.

However, if you do continue to feel discomfort when feeding, do not hesitate to refer to your *resource list* to find the support you need. If you are still in hospital, ask midwives to observe a feed, or ask whether a lactation consultant is available. If you are at home, it is a good idea to go through the steps of attachment earlier in this book (Chapter 5) and also later in this chapter. When your nipples are in the correct position in baby's mouth, even if sore or damaged, you will notice an immediate improvement. You will also notice that baby feeds more efficiently, detaching by himself when he has had enough and leaving your nipple in its pre-feed shape.

Think carefully about what you feel as your baby feeds. If it doesn't feel right, remove him gently from your breast by slipping your finger into the side of his mouth and down onto his lower gum to break the suction. Remove your nipple, readjust yourself ensuring that you are in your most comfortable position, and start again. If feeding remains uncomfortable or your nipples are very sore, contact who you think is the most appropriate for help. In the meantime, if possible, continue to breastfeed, paying particular attention to positioning and attachment. After feeds, express a little breastmilk to cover your nipples and areola and air dry them before replacing your bra. This is the best first aid treatment but the important thing is to take action early.

There may be other reasons for sore nipples:

- Baby has been having bottles and is sucking on your breast as if it was the teat of a bottle. Early use of a dummy can have the same effect. It can cause nipple confusion, as the sucking on a teat is very different than suckling at the breast.

- **Tongue-tie**. When nipples are persistently sore despite all measures to maximise baby's positioning and attachment to the breast, it is worth checking baby's mouth. A tongue-tie relates to the narrow strip of skin that attaches the tongue to the bottom of the mouth. It is called the *frenulum*. Usually, it is no problem, except when it connects too far forward onto the tongue, sometimes distorting its shape at the tip. It may also be unusually thick. Baby's tongue is essential for efficient feeding because it needs to wrap around your nipple and part of the areola, to draw breastmilk in a rhythmic action to swallow. When tongue-tie is severe enough, it restricts this movement, making feeding painful and ineffective.

Sometimes this is overlooked—or baby's mouth is checked for a tongue-tie problem, but is not accurately diagnosed. This is very frustrating for parents. An undiagnosed tongue-tie can cause other breastfeeding problems, the main one, apart from mother discomfort, being a reduced transfer of milk from mother to baby. This can lead to weight gain issues, as well as an unsettled baby... and stress.

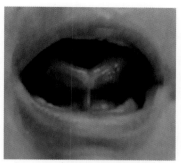

A more easily recognisable tongue-tie

An International Board Certified Lactation Consultant (IBCLC) or a doctor familiar with babies can check baby's mouth accurately and refer you to appropriate action by a paediatric dentist or orofacial surgeon. Treatment can be simple—the frenulum can be snipped or severed by a laser. Usually, it is quick with little blood loss and can be followed with a soothing breastfeed.

- **Thrush**: Bothersome thrush is caused by a very normal and common fungus called *Candida Albicans*. This generally lives happily in our bodies until for some reason its balance is upset. Babies are usually introduced to it at birth, or soon after. This balance can be disturbed by the use of antibiotics, which destroys good bacteria, but not the fungus organism. In doing so, the thrush has room to flourish. You could suspect thrush if :

  - your nipples become sore after a period of pain-free nursing
  - baby has a nappy rash that isn't responding to normal healing creams (the rash is reddish, with red dots around the edges)

- baby has white patches on his tongue that can't be wiped off. When it is more advanced, you may notice white spots or patches on the inside of baby's lips and cheeks

- you have had in the past, a course of antibiotics and your nipples are sore or very sensitive

Thrush needs to be treated, because if it is left to develop, you may notice that as well as sore nipples, pain may be felt deep in your breast, even continuing after you have finished feeding. Baby may be particularly *fussy* when feeding, attaching and detaching frequently. Treatment usually consists of an antifungal medication both in baby's mouth and on your nipples after feeds, four times a day. This can be bought without a prescription from most pharmacies and usually works very well. But treatment does need to be continued for at least four days after symptoms have resolved. It is helpful to have a GP who is familiar with breastfeeding and able to diagnose this condition accurately.

- **Raynaud's syndrome**: A small number of mothers experience this, making feeding unpleasant and painful. It is a sudden blanching of nipples, usually after baby has fed. It is accompanied by a burning sensation when circulation returns and blood vessels open up again. Nipples become quite red, often throbbing with pain before returning to their usual pinkness. Sometimes Raynaud's syndrome is associated with other causes of nipple soreness, like thrush or poor attachment. Treating possible causes may resolve symptoms. Strategies that may help are keeping breasts warm with heat packs before and after feeds and cutting down or eliminating smoking (smoking can affect circulation). Fish oil capsules have been known to help some women. If Raynaud's syndrome continues to be a problem, investigate further with the help of your GP. A medication called Nifedipine is occasionally used and may help to relieve symptoms.

How to manage feeding discomfort regardless of the cause

Firstly, consider contacting someone appropriate on your *resource list* for assessment of your particular situation. Early action is important. Breastfeeding should be comfortable and relaxing. You can also review the steps below for attachment, as the way baby latches, affects what you are feeling. Also, correct attachment affects the transfer of your milk as baby feeds, so it is of vital importance.

- Review the attachment diagrams in Chapter 5

- Ensure you are comfortable before you feed (toilet, drink etc.)

- Skin-to-skin if possible will enhance baby's natural feeding instincts

- Start on the least sore side

- As you hold baby close, his tummy to your tummy, gently express a little milk for him to smell

- Let your breast fall into its natural position, bringing baby to breast, not breast to baby

- Have your arm along his back, with your open hand at the top of his shoulders—not touching his head

- Have your nipple pointing to his top lip and his head slightly extended, so his chin and bottom lip come to your breast first. This is important

- As his chin comes into your breast and with it his bottom lip, the touch will stimulate him to open his mouth widely, with his tongue in the correct position for feeding

- Observe, and at this precise moment, use your hand at the top of his shoulders to very firmly bring him straight into your breast. It may look as if his chin is burrowing into your breast first, with his two cheeks and nose also firmly touching. This is normal. In this position, he can draw in your nipple and a large part of the areola and take it to the back part of his mouth where the soft part of his palate is. You should feel no pain— but let baby have eight to ten sucks as you assess how it feels.

- Do not worry that his nose appears to be partly blocked by your breast. Baby's noses are designed to let air in and a quarter of a nostril will be enough for this. If concerned, you can bring his nose more off your breast, by using your arm, or the elbow part of your arm, to bring his bottom closer into your body. This has the effect of extending his head a little more, thus lifting his nose back.

Nipple shields

If sore nipples are not resolving and you are feeling distressed by feeding discomfort, you may be advised to use a nipple shield as a short-term helper. A nipple shield is a silicone cover that is positioned over your nipple during feeding. This may sound an easy solution, but because of less direct stimulation, breasts may not be emptied as efficiently, which can eventually lead to a fall in milk supply. Additionally, baby may prefer the nipple shield and may be reluctant to re-attach directly to the breast when nipples are less sore. Nipple shields can be useful, but use them with caution and don't hesitate to seek support to re-attach baby directly to your breast as soon as possible. If using a nipple shield, it is a good idea to seek advice from a lactation consultant, who can support you and baby back to breastfeeding without it when nipples are less sore.

If you have developed unbearably painful or damaged nipples, as a last resort (when everything else has been tried), you may decide, or you may be advised, to cease feeding baby at the breast for a short time to allow for healing. This period will vary, depending on your situation; a few feeds or perhaps twenty-four hours, before recommencing breastfeeding. In such case, you will need to consider firstly, expression of your breastmilk and secondly, the best way for you to give it to your baby.

Expressing

It is useful to know about breastmilk expression for short-term situations as in the above case. As time goes on, and once learned, expressing can be used for a variety of situations, making feeding more flexible. It is particularly relevant if you are considering a return to work.

The main ways to express are either by hand or using a breast pump. Although expensive, people generally find the high-grade electric pumps most effective. Hand expression costs nothing and with practice can become easy and efficient. Some mothers may already be familiar with hand expression if they followed the *antenatal expression of colostrum* regime described in Chapter 2.

How to hand express

If you refer back to the breast diagram in Chapter 1, you can see how the milk ducts that form a circle around your breast all lead towards the nipple area. The ducts are most concentrated just behind the darker skin of the areola. The area around the areola needs gentle, rhythmic pressure to eject milk. (You can see why baby needs a wide-open mouth when attaching to feed!)

Firstly, make sure you are warm, comfortable and relaxed, which is often easier when you are in a private situation. You need clean hands and a wide-mouthed container that has been rinsed with boiling water. Encourage a *let down* by gently massaging your breasts towards your nipples, working around the whole breast.

Place your thumb on the top of your areola where it meets the rest of your breast and your forefinger in the opposite position underneath. Gently press your fingers back towards your ribs, feeling the main part of your breast tissue between your fingers. Firmly compress your fingers together with a rolling forward action. This has the effect of compressing the milk ducts, pushing the milk out without hurting sensitive breast tissue.

Continue this action rhythmically until the *let down* occurs, which may take a few minutes. Your milk will eject either in a spray or a dribble, (or maybe just one or two drops if it is colostrum). Continue this action until the flow of milk slows, ⍺

and finger position to another part of ⍵

around the areola with these rhythmic

Avoid squeezing your breast as this

pulling on your nipple, as this can ⍳

pressure. You⍳

attaches to⍳

cause yo⍳

irrita⍳

yo⍳

When the amount of milk you can express ᵣₒₘ

breast decreases, change to the other breast and repeat the proc⍳

You can go back and forth between breasts until you have the required amount of milk. Change hands if they become tired. Do not let your fingers slip on your breasts as this can irritate and damage your skin, so have a cloth handy to dry your hands as you move the position of your fingers. Also, do not be discouraged if you do not get much milk—it is not an indication of how much milk you have. It often takes much practice before hand expression becomes really easy and fast.

Using an electric pump

There is a variety of breast pumps on the market, particularly since many women continue to breastfeed after returning to work. The choice of the pump will depend on the reasons for needing to express. Electric pumps are expensive but can be hired from pharmacies or from your local breastfeeding resource group. In Australia, it is the ABA or Australian Breastfeeding Association. Some Lactation Consultants working in private practice hire out breast pumps and will ensure that the parts of the pump fit your breasts and function appropriately. Ideally, a breast pump should create a good seal with adjustable suction

nipple needs to be centred in the flange that
your breast so that the rhythmic suction does not
ur nipples to rub against the sides. This would further
e sore nipples. Again, when using any pump, it is easier if
u are warm, relaxed and in a private or comfortable setting.
You will find additional information about expressing and
storing breastmilk included in Chapter 11.

How much does baby need for a feed?

Babies take differing amounts at feed times—there is a wide
feed-to-feed variability, so it is difficult to know how much to aim
to have for each feed. Consequently, it is wise if possible to have
small amounts, for example, 50ml of expressed breastmilk stored
in the fridge or freezer, so that wastage of your precious milk is
minimal. This is especially so if the reason you are expressing is
short term. More can be offered without wastage.

Taking this into account, a very general guide for how much milk
is needed depends on the age and weight of baby. Baby needs
approximately 180ml of breastmilk per kilogram of body weight
within twenty-four hours. This amount can be divided by the
average number of feeds in that time.

An example of this is:

Baby has an average of 8 feeds in 24 hours and weighs 4 kilograms.
180ml x 4 kilograms = 720ml
Divide 720ml by 8 feeds = 90 ml per feed

How to give the expressed milk to your baby

If you need to feed expressed milk to your baby in the early days or weeks, it is better to avoid using a bottle if possible. This is because of the different sucking action needed when using an artificial teat, which can confuse baby and make re-attachment to the breast more difficult. If baby is in hospital, as could be the case if baby is premature, midwives and medical staff will guide you according to your particular situation.

Cup feeding: Expressed breastmilk can be given to a young baby efficiently via a small cup. It does not seem to interfere with breastfeeding and baby gets the nourishment he needs during the time that he cannot, for whatever reason, feed directly from the breast. To do this, have your milk in a medicine cup or small shot glass and your baby sitting on your knee in a fairly upright position, with his head supported. It may help to have baby wrapped in a light cotton sheet to avoid arms knocking and spilling precious milk supplies. Place the cup on his lower gums and gently tilt the cup, and the baby, back a little until he tastes some milk on his tongue. You will then see him start to bring his tongue forward and lap the milk. The first time you do it may seem awkward, but with practice, it becomes easier.

Finger feeding: Another way to give baby milk short-term so as not to interfere with breastfeeding attachment is by *finger feeding*. This method requires you to have a thin plastic or rubber tube that has one end in a bottle or container of milk and the other end taped or held alongside the middle finger of your right or left hand—whichever feels most comfortable.

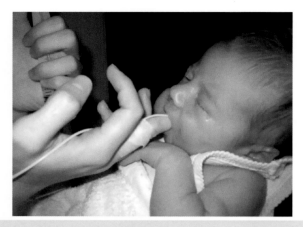

The tubing that is generally used is part of a 'Supplementary Nursing System' or 'Supply line', that can be purchased from breastfeeding support agencies such as the Australian Breastfeeding Association. The system is further discussed in Chapter 8.

Ensure that your fingernail is short and, of course, that your hands are well-washed and clean. As baby sucks, let him draw your finger (and the tube) to the back of his mouth, preferably to where his soft palate starts and up to your second knuckle. This depends on your hand size. Have your finger upturned, so that the pad is uppermost in baby's mouth, and straight so that his tongue is kept flat and forward. This is more like feeding at your breast than if baby was feeding via the teat of a bottle. As baby sucks, he is using more of his face and jaw muscles than if he was bottle feeding, and the milk can be drawn quite efficiently through the tube.

Note: When baby is older, with breastfeeding firmly established and gaining weight, occasionally feeding expressed breastmilk

Low milk supply—not enough milk?

Many factors can contribute to low milk supply, but most often it is related to baby not feeding well from the breast. Fix the feeding problem, and breastmilk supply will inevitably improve. Some situations make this extra challenging, for example when a baby is born prematurely or is sick; when mother is unwell; or if there has been a prolonged mother/baby separation after birth. Other situations can make it particularly difficult to produce enough milk, and these cases are discussed fully in Chapter 8. Most women, even in poor countries where undernutrition is a concern, can produce enough milk for their babies. (Newman, 2006). Inability to produce milk or enough milk is rare.

Sometimes, milk supply can be perceived as being low when in actual fact it is okay.

If for some reason baby is crying and unsettled it can diminish confidence and increase parents' stress levels. It may lead to thoughts that insufficient milk supply is the cause of the problem. Confidence is important, and knowledge leads to confidence. This is not the time to offer a bottle of formula, to watch baby guzzle it down, impacting on your belief that you haven't enough milk.

For a baby who attaches well and feeds often enough, a low milk supply should not be an issue. The more milk that baby takes, the more is made. Ideally, baby feeds whenever and as often as he needs to be—baby-led, not clock-led. If this is happening, your baby should be gaining weight and showing other positive signs in his general development that his food intake is adequate.

On the other hand, a baby that has not learnt from early days to attach and suckle successfully may not be stimulating your breasts in the way needed to make enough milk. Additionally, you may be experiencing nipple soreness or pain because of the way the baby is suckling. Your nipple might be rubbing up against the roof of his mouth as he feeds, rather than being further back in the soft palate. Feeds maybe taking a long time, and you may have a crying unsettled baby. This can make you tired and stressed as you try to work it all out. And, on top of all this, you may have well-meaning family or friends confusing you with their advice— all reducing your confidence and self-esteem. No wonder a *quick fix bottle of formula* looks attractive.

Low milk supply or a perceived low milk supply is a major reason women cease breastfeeding.

To help work out whether you have a genuine concern or not, ask yourself:

- Is our baby looking healthy?

- Does baby have six or more wet nappies a day?

- Are baby's bowel actions soft and is he having at least one a day in the early weeks?

- Am I feeding often enough during the day, and at least once during the night?

- Is baby going through a phase of being extra hungry? Is baby experiencing a growth surge?

- What is the overall trend of his weight, length and head circumference? (Check growth charts in baby's health record)

Most importantly, ask yourself what else is going on in your life? Am I eating and can I sleep well when I get a chance? These are some things you may like to discuss with your health professional or someone on your *resource list*.

If your uneasiness continues, tap into your *resource list* early. Do not leave it to crisis point. Do not hesitate to ask for support loudly and confidently. The problem may not be resulting from poor attachment, and the situation needs to be looked at holistically. For example, your baby may be unwell, appearing sleepy and uninterested in feeding, and therefore *telling* your breasts to not make as much milk. Baby's growth may, as a result, be static or even dropping. This is a situation that needs prompt attention so that you can receive guidance as to what you need to do to attend to baby's health, as well as increase your milk supply. Usually, the best thing you can do is to keep breastfeeding and follow specific advice given by a trusted professional.

Be wary of any advice, whatever the source, that suggests baby be given bottles. Do seek a second opinion. An International Board Certified Lactation Consultant (IBCLC) would be an excellent choice. I have experienced many situations where breastfeeding progress has been ruined by the unnecessary introduction of formula from a bottle. When formula is introduced unnecessarily, your breasts are 'told' not to make as much milk. Breasts have less stimulation. The formula remains in the baby's body for longer because it digests less easily than breastmilk. Therefore baby does not demand a feed as often,

As mentioned earlier, it may be you think your milk supply is low because of baby's behaviour. It can be quite common for baby to go through unsettled periods, when he is particularly hungry and demanding. It may be that he needs a little more milk at this time for growing. Or perhaps he needs more close suckling time with you. Feeding more often and offering a *top up* breastfeed if he seems to want more after his usual feed, will often satisfy him. Additionally, this is great stimulation for your milk supply.

Generally, if you are concerned about your milk supply, the first line of treatment after baby's health is assessed, is to pay close attention to baby's attachment and suckling. Improvement can make a marked difference in the amount of milk you are making. This is because of the stimulation of the of the nerves around your nipples and areola when baby is actively feeding. These nerves communicate with your brain, which in turn sends messages to the breast to *make more milk*.

As mentioned before, the natural hormones oxytocin and prolactin play a significant part—the more those hormones are activated, the more milk is made. The hormones are best activated by baby suckling. So the second line of treatment is to encourage baby to feed more frequently. This may mean that for a few days you aim to feed as often as possible. Skin-to-skin contact will help encourage baby's natural feeding instincts. If time and energy allow, it may be appropriate to express your milk in frequent short sessions after baby has fed. This can also have the effect of building up supply.

Keep a general eye on baby's overall weight progress. If you plot baby's weight on the graph in your baby's Health Record over a period of time, you will usually see a gradual upward trend along a percentile line somewhere between the 3rd and 97th percentile. Use this as just one tool to assess whether your baby is getting enough milk.

Other useful strategies may involve stopping dummy or pacifier use (if you are using one), so that baby has only one way of sucking for comfort and food—on the breast. This gives maximum stimulation for milk production.

Medications called *galactagogues* can be useful when all other strategies for increasing milk supply have been considered. One that is commonly prescribed is Domperidone, which works by increasing the levels of the milk-making hormone, prolactin. If using this or any other galactagogue, do so with a medically supervised plan according to your particular situation.

Because *perceived insufficient breastmilk* is the number one reason in many countries that formula is introduced, to the detriment of breastfeeding longevity, I'll include with permission, this segment from the website www.kellymom.com. (K, Bonyata 2017).

Is your milk supply really low?

If your baby is gaining weight and having an adequate amount of wet nappies, you *do not* have a low milk supply.

The following *do not* indicate a low supply:

- baby nurses frequently

- baby suddenly increases the frequency or length of nursing sessions (cluster feeding)

- baby nurses more often and is fussy in the evenings

- baby frequently wakes in the night

- baby doesn't nurse as long as previously

- baby guzzles down a bottle of expressed milk or formula after a nursing session

- your breasts suddenly seem softer

- your breasts don't leak anymore

- you stop feeling, or never felt a *let down* sensation

- you get very little or no milk while expressing

Slow Weight Gain

The issue of slow weight gain in a baby can go hand in hand with low milk supply. Improving one will often have the effect of enhancing the other. Of course, it is important that the baby's general health and development is reviewed by an appropriate health professional as a slow weight gain could be due to baby being unwell.

A useful way to increase baby's weight and increase milk supply is to adopt a temporary daytime pattern with baby. When feeding, offer both sides if possible and follow with a short *playtime*. Then offer another quick feed, like a *top-up*, before settling for sleep. This may sound complicated, but it is really quite simple. The following explains how this strategy can be used.

- Taking care with attachment, let baby feed on the first side until he comes off satisfied having finished *the first breast first.*

- After a brief break, perhaps a nappy change or cuddle over your shoulder (remembering that extensive *burping* is not necessary), offer and encourage feeding from your second breast.

- When finished, even though he might be quite sleepy, try a *play* on the floor. This involves eye contact, talking, singing, stroking and playing. Babies will often become more awake and enjoy this time very much, with movements being relaxed and hands more unclenched than clenched. He will look at you and *talk* with you.

- After a short time (depending on the age of your baby), you will notice some tired signs developing. The main ones for a very young baby are clenched fists, jerkier type movements, facial grimace, and a grizzle. You may also notice less direct eye contact.

- At this point, pick him up and offer a short feed from the side you finished on. He may have some from the other breast as well. Try to keep this second brief *top-up* feed within an hour of the beginning of the main feed.

- Repeat this pattern during his day feeds, (not during the night) and continue until weight gain and supply are improving.

If your health professional has suggested that it is necessary for baby to have additional nutrition to boost his weight, an efficient way to do this without compromising breastfeeding is with the help of a *Supplemental Nursing System,* or *supply-line.* This consists of a fine plastic tube, one end taped to the breast and the other attached to a container of milk. This is an effective way to boost baby's intake, while also encouraging him to feed at the breast and stimulate milk production.

Supplemental Nursing System or 'supply line'

This can be a useful tool because not only does baby get extra food, he has to suckle at the breast to receive it, thus stimulating milk production. Baby gets the extra milk via the tube that is taped to your breast, the tip of which protrudes slightly out from your nipple. A container holding your milk can be positioned around your neck via a soft cord. It is particularly helpful that baby receives extra milk via the breast because he has less chance of being confused by foreign bottle teats in his mouth that require a different type of sucking. The supplementary milk can be formula but expressed breastmilk is preferable. To get started with this, support from a lactation consultant or midwife who is familiar with this way of feeding would be valuable.

Initially, it can be quite fiddly to manipulate everything—the 'supply line' tubing, the extra milk in position, and maybe a wriggling baby in arms. Some mothers find it easier than others. Usually, it helps if you get everything ready beforehand—milk in a container, tape cut prepared for when the tubing is placed in position and ideally, someone to assist. With practice and patience, it can become a short-term routine that is easily handled.

When using this strategy to supplement baby's intake, take care to position and attach him to the breast correctly so that he receives the maximum amount of milk as he suckles, as well as extra via the tubing. The method can be used for as long as is necessary. The aim is to reduce the amount he has via the *supply line*, as his weight and your milk production increase.

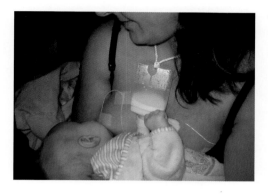

Engorgement

Usually, on the third or fourth day after baby is born, hormones cause your breasts to fill with extra fluid, (not just milk) making them feel full and firm. This can be even more so if intravenous fluids (a drip) have been used during labour. Normally, this fullness subsides within the first weeks. The discomfort can be avoided or minimalised by encouraging baby to feed frequently, aiming to *empty* one breast as fully as possible each time you feed. Keeping baby for as long as he will stay on the first breast, before offering the second, helps with this. Warm compresses can be used before feeds to help the flow of milk, and cold compresses can be used between feeds to ease discomfort. If extreme, just once, it may be helpful to express your milk as completely as possible. An electric pump would be ideal for this. *Emptying* as much as you can, assists the drainage of the extra fluids that have settled in breast tissue. Another treatment that seems to have a soothing effect is positioning green cabbage leaves over your breasts underneath your bra for about twenty minutes several times a day (Mohrbacher, 2012).

The danger of prolonged engorgement is that it leads to milk and fluid in your breasts not moving much, or being static. This may give the wrong feedback messages to your body's milk-making mechanisms. It also could lead to baby having difficulty latching, even eventually causing inflammation of breast tissue leading to mastitis (more about mastitis in Chapter 7). Usually, with early frequent breastfeeds with baby attaching well, engorged breasts are not a problem.

Too much milk, or oversupply

Even though initial *engorgement* subsides, there are a few women who are particularly good at producing milk and progress on to produce copious amounts—far more than their baby needs: an oversupply. There may also be a fast *let-down*, which causes baby to become uncomfortable feeding. He may cough, choke and splutter, pulling back from the breast as he feeds, trying to cope with the fast flow of milk. He can be windy and unsettled, have a *rumbly tummy* and frothy, sometimes *explosive*, bowel actions. Usually, this problem regulates itself in time, as baby's milk requirement balances the amount of milk made.

Fast flow

If you do experience a particularly fast flow of your milk at the beginning of feeds that is overwhelming for baby, you may find these strategies help.

• Gently massage breasts before feeds to start the let-down reflex. Catch this more forceful milk in a cloth. When baby attaches to feed, the flow will have slowed.

- Or, have baby attach and start suckling. As soon as the milk starts flowing in a rush, gently remove baby and catch the *fast milk* in a cloth. When it slows after a few seconds, reattach baby to your breast to continue the feed.

- Try using the *laid back* or *biological nursing* position to feed baby as demonstrated in Chapter 5. This allows baby to be higher than your breast when feeding and gives him more control over a fast let-down.

- As baby gets bigger and more able to cope with the flow, you can momentarily place an outstretched finger across the top or side of your breast to slow the flow a fraction, just while the let-down is occurring. This may be all that is needed.

If oversupply does not settle and is causing you and baby distress these temporary strategies may help. It is always worth having baby's feeding assessed by an appropriate health professional before trying to change your production of milk. If trying these strategies, be alert to breast changes, for example, redness or soreness, that could indicate impending inflammation, or mastitis.

- One breast per feed. Let baby finish the first side before offering the same breast for the last part of the feed. This will encourage your milk supply to reduce to meet his need. Ensure that you start the next feed on the other side.

- If baby is unsettled and *colicky*, offer him the same breast for several feeds. The other breast can be offered for the next few feeds. This is sometimes called *block-feeding*. This also encourages his intake of the higher calorie *hindmilk*, which slows his gut down and makes him feel fuller for longer and therefore less windy or colicky. This strategy will also help your milk supply to reduce. At any time a breast is feeling too full, express just a little for comfort.

Always be careful with positioning and attaching baby correctly so that each breast has the best chance of being emptied regularly. Avoid breasts becoming overfull or sore. Full breasts are more susceptible to blocked ducts and mastitis.

Mastitis

Mastitis is a reasonably common, unpleasant obstacle that is usually caused when breastmilk builds up unevenly in your breasts, leading to stasis or lack of movement. If left untreated, it can quickly develop into a full-blown infection that may need antibiotic treatment. In the early stages, you will often notice a painful red area on your breast. Left to progress, you may feel general aches and pains and have an elevated temperature, with flu-like symptoms.

Mastitis is caused by any interruption to your milk flow—such as a tight bra, clothes pulling tightly into your armpit when feeding, or baby changing the frequency of his feeding. It seems to affect women more if they are tired and run down and can start quite suddenly. Because of this, it is valuable to know about mastitis, what to do to avoid it and how to treat it if it occurs.

Most people will never experience mastitis, but there is no harm in being one step ahead by being aware of how your breasts feel and look.

To avoid the possibility of mastitis, it is a good idea to:

- Check your breasts each day—when you have a shower is as good a time as any. Gently feel around each breast to check if you have any tender areas. Lactating breasts may feel quite *lumpy*, but shouldn't have any sore, red or very tender areas.

- When you wear bras, ensure they are supportive, not tight and that they don't have seams or wires that dig in or irritate your breasts in any way.

- When feeding, especially in the early months, take care in how you hold and latch baby onto your breast. Always remove baby and start again if it doesn't feel comfortable. Do this by placing your small finger into the side of baby's mouth, with gentle downward pressure on bottom gums to break the suction. Nipples that are damaged due to incorrect attachment are susceptible to bacteria entering into milk ducts, possibly leading to mastitis.

- Alternate the side that you start on, letting baby feed until satisfied before offering the other side That is, finish the first breast first. That way, each breast has a regular emptying.

Try not to let yourself get run down, which means it is really important that you eat and drink well—every day, (not just to avoid mastitis). Sleep and rest are essential. From early days, be kind to yourself; go slowly where you can and if possible, factor in regular rest time. Importantly, accept help from trusted family or friends without feeling guilty about it. Say, 'Yes, that would be great', rather than 'No, we're fine thanks'.

Treating mastitis

Mastitis can be stopped in its tracks if caught in the early stages.

You may notice a sore red patch on a part of your breast. That breast needs to be drained well to stop any blockage progressing. Feed on that sore side first to encourage emptying.

- Before feeding, you can place a moderately warm compress over the area to stimulate blood circulation. This relieves discomfort and encourages the movement of milk.

- Between feeds, a cold compress over the affected area can feel soothing and reduce swelling.

- You can also gently massage from behind the sensitive area down towards your nipple. The skin on your breasts is very delicate. When massaging, a tiny bit of an organic oil will help your fingers slide, rather than drag and stretch your skin.

- If possible, as baby is feeding, you can gently massage the sensitive area to help mobilise milk that may be banked up in milk ducts.

- Additionally, if it is possible, have baby's chin pointing towards this area. When baby feeds, ideally his chin is well into your breast. (see diagrams in Chapter 5). The movement of his jaw naturally massages the area, thus helping with milk flow. This may mean that you change baby's feeding position to the football or under arm hold, as opposed to the more usual cradle hold.

- If baby only takes one side, it may be that the other breast feels overfull and uncomfortable. In this case, you will need to express milk to ensure that that breast does not develop problems.

It is not always possible to get in early and treat mastitis in this way. For example, baby may have changed his feeding pattern, sleeping more during the night. You may wake in the morning and with little or no warning feel unwell with general aches, pains and sore breasts. This can quickly progress to mastitis. Regardless of the cause, there are things you can do to turn the situation around.

- It is most important to keep breastfeeding to encourage regular breast emptying, and baby suckling is the best way to do this. Your milk is still perfect—the only difference is that it may taste a little salty during the time you have mastitis, which baby will adjust to. Feeding lying down sideways in bed if you are feeling unwell may be helpful.

- An analgesic, such as Panadol, can ease discomfort and reduce fever.

- Some parents make an appointment with their doctor for later in the day, just in case symptoms are not diminishing, and then cancel if the situation is improving.

- Antibiotics, work very well and usually reverse the symptoms of mastitis within twenty-four hours. This is where it is useful to have the backup of a medical appointment to get an accurate diagnosis and if necessary, a prescription for an appropriate antibiotic.

A blocked duct

A blocked milk duct is experienced as a local sore area, often, but not always, with a white *bleb* or blister on your nipple. The discomfort is caused by fat globules clogging the flow, with milk banking up behind. So, as with mastitis, it is the result of part of your breast not being drained properly. It does differ in that it often resolves as baby breastfeeds. Instant relief is sometimes experienced if, following a warm compress on the area, the outer skin on the *bleb* is lifted with a sterile needle and baby is fed—ideally with his chin pointing to the sore area. This may mean changing your usual feeding position to one that facilitates this. You can also try massaging the area towards the nipple after the warm compress and hand expressing, even gently squeezing the blocked duct to encourage it to clear, before feeding baby. You may find that a *string* of thickish material comes out of the duct, giving you reasonably quick relief.

An unresolved blocked duct can progress to mastitis and even a breast abscess requiring medical diagnosis and antibiotics. If symptoms do not improve with the above treatment, please seek further appropriate help. Again, refer to your *resource list*. This may also mean reviewing baby's positioning and feeding technique so that optimal drainage is encouraged.

Reflux

It is common and quite normal for young babies to bring up small amounts of milk, usually after feeds. This does not worry babies in the slightest. It happens because the muscle or valve at the top of young babies stomaches is not as efficient or mature as it will be when older. It usually becomes more toned by four months. Instead of contracting and holding milk in baby's stomach to digest, the muscle allows it to move up and down the food pipe (the *oesophagus*) freely. Sometimes it is re-swallowed, but often it spills out causing wet, milky patches on shoulders and laps.

It only turns into a problem when it becomes more regular, happening well after the feed has finished. This is when, because it is mixed with the baby's acidic stomach juices, the oesophagus eventually becomes irritated and sore. This causes baby to cry with discomfort, which, of course, is distressing for parents, as well as for baby. This is when it is called *gastric reflux,* or *gastro-oesophageal reflux.*

Useful suggestions if 'spilling' is causing a problem

- Obtain an accurate diagnosis by a professional who listens well to your explanation of baby's symptoms. Depending on the severity you may be advised to start medication that reduces the acidity in baby's stomach and helps food to pass through more quickly, away from his top stomach muscle.

However, usually, reflux can be managed without medication.

In a few situations, milk spills are more like larger vomits, that could be related to allergy or intolerance. Because baby will have tiny percentages of what you eat and drink, occasionally it is advised that you try not eating certain things (for example, dairy products) to see if it makes a difference.

- Calm baby if he is upset before you start feeding. If baby is calm and relaxed, he is less likely to vomit.

- Feed baby for as long as he will stay on your breast at each feed. When he is feeding/swallowing, there are downward waves of muscular contractions (called *peristalsis*) along his oesophagus and stomach, encouraging food to pass through and away from that top stomach muscle. While this is happening, the acidic stomach juices mixed with milk will not come back and trouble him.

- One of the advantages of breastmilk is that it is easily and relatively quickly digested, so it passes through baby's system promptly. Ultrasound studies have shown that a baby's stomach filled with breastmilk empties in thirty-five minutes (Chilton, 2013). Formula, which is more difficult to digest, remains in the stomach for longer, possibly causing more intense reflux.

- While baby is awake after a feed, cuddle him in a more upright position. A baby sling is perfect as it keeps him close and upright. Gravity helps keep the stomach contents away from the top stomach muscle. This is fine for a small baby but can be tiring as he grows heavier.

- Avoid having his nappy done up too firmly, as this could put pressure on his stomach, which in turn could put pressure on the top stomach muscle.

Colic

Colic is a common complaint that can stress parents as they try to work out the cause of prolonged bouts of crying for no apparent reason. Baby may draw up his knees as if he has a tummy ache and screw up his face. He is often fussy when feeding and unhappy afterwards, even though he is gaining weight and progressing well developmentally. It is most common in the evenings, perhaps when parents are more tired and less able to cope. It often starts around four weeks of age and thankfully, subsides by three months. Parents try everything to soothe and comfort baby and are often bamboozled by the cause. So it is understandable that they start to think that maybe it is the breastmilk or breastfeeding that is causing the behaviour. Confidence can be undermined. Switching to formula will not help to resolve the issue and doing so deprives the baby of all the breastfeeding advantages.

Colic coping strategies

- Firstly, try to stay calm as parents' tension can be sensed by baby, making the situation worse.

- Holding, cuddling, talking and stroking will help calm and reassure baby, even as he is crying. It is never okay to let him *cry it out*, or ignore his cries. It is his only means of communication with you, and by promptly responding to him you are laying the important foundations of trust and feelings of safety.

- When feeding, always ensure that he is attached well and it feels comfortable for you. Encourage him to finish the first breast first, before offering the other side. This is so he has plenty of the creamier *hindmilk* towards the end of the feed. This helps to slow his gut down, making him feel fuller for longer. It is higher in calories than the first part of the feed, the *foremilk*.

- For a few feeds, you can try putting him back to the first breast for the second part of his feed to encourage this hindmilk intake. Sometimes in the early weeks, baby fills up with the first part of the feed, which contains thirst quenching and satisfying milk, but is higher in lactose or sugar. As it is digested, it can cause baby to feel windy or colicky. If this is the case, you may also notice baby has frequent *explosive* bowel actions.

Beware of anyone suggesting that your baby is 'lactose intolerant' at this time. True lactose intolerance is extremely rare.

- A warm bath can be very soothing and calming, as can gentle tummy massage in a clockwise direction; the same direction as the large intestine.

- If colic continues to be a problem after trying these strategies, as well as using your *resource list* for information and support, it is wise to have your baby's health checked by a doctor or paediatrician. It can be reassuring to know that there is nothing that you have overlooked and that symptoms will decrease as baby grows.

How to manage breastfeeding with large breasts

The size of your breasts does not mean *more milk* or *less milk*. All breasts, large or small, except in rare cases, produce all the milk that your baby needs—and more. This is providing baby attaches well and feeds frequently enough. Particularly large breasts can influence breastfeeding because it can be more difficult to position baby to feed comfortably. It can be harder to view what is going on when baby is attaching. Some ideas to help with this are:

- To lift your breast so it is in a better position for you to see, place a rolled up nappy or small towel under your breast.

- Have baby positioned level with your nipple and areola. You may find pillows are useful for support—although you may find that your lap gives all the support that is needed.

- Experiment with different positions. Side-lying or with

baby under your arm in the footy hold is a popular, comfortable position.

- Breastfeeding in front of a mirror. This will give you a different and hopefully helpful view of baby attaching.

- When attaching baby to feed, try using a 'breast sandwich' to make a firm area that is his mouth size. To do this, compress breast with fingers above and below, well back from the areola. As baby opens his mouth to attach, bring him into you firmly, with his chin leading the way and his head slightly tilted back. Once he has attached and is suckling, remove your hand, and relax. Remember, he only needs part of a nostril to breath properly as he feeds.

- Larger breasts can be heavy and become hot, so a good supportive bra—one that is of an absorbent cotton material without underwires, is ideal.

- Feeding when out and about can feel daunting at first, regardless of breast size. Remember, that feeding your baby wherever you are is the most natural thing in the world. It is legal everywhere to feed in public. It is what you should do. If self-conscious, you can use a light scarf or sheet to cover your upper body as baby feeds.

But just do it! Breastfeeding in public will become easier and easier if you do.

Postnatal depression

I include postnatal depression here because it is reasonably common in the first year after baby is born and can have a considerable impact on the way a mother feels about herself and her baby. It can take the joy out of parenthood and damage the breastfeeding relationship. It can impact both parents.

Earlier I touched on the issue of *the third-day blues* which frequently occur three to four days after baby is born. It is a low feeling after the euphoria of baby's birth, and occurs in approximately 80% of mothers. It is usually short-lived, lasting a few days. You may feel quite suddenly overwhelmed and teary. It is thought to be caused by a dramatic shift in natural hormones that assist your body in returning to its non-pregnant state. It sometimes causes emotional upheaval in the process. This type of *dip* or lowering of emotional state is quite normal and disappears after a day or two without needing any treatment apart from understanding and support.

If these low feelings persist for more than two weeks, there is a chance that they will develop into mild or moderate postnatal depression. Mothers experience this differently, but common symptoms include constant anxiety, inability to relax or sleep and therefore extreme tiredness. Sometimes mothers will say they have a reduced appetite for food, dramatic mood swings and feelings of low self-worth. (Riordan and Wambach, 2010).

Generally, when breastfeeding is going well, your risk of postnatal depression is lowered. (Mohrbacher, 2012) This is partly because of the influence of the oxytocin hormone, which reduces stress levels and induces relaxed, sleepy states as you feed. Regardless, it still occurs in some women, influenced by factors such as isolation and the overwhelming responsibility of managing a new baby. It is important to **act early** if you do have any persisting symptoms. Postnatal depression can affect your relationship with your baby, your partner, breastfeeding and your general health. It may feel daunting to make the first step in asking for help or advice - your close support people may be the best to advocate for you. In most communities, there are active support services and GPs. Or you may have specific contacts on your *resource list*. It often helps enormously to talk freely about how you are honestly feeling while continuing to nourish and comfort your baby with breastfeeds as you move through this period. If needed, medications compatible with breastfeeding can be prescribed and can help immensely.

In addition to talking to the appropriate people and following the recommended treatment, many women have reported that physical exercise can be especially helpful when combating depression. A brisk daily walk, ideally in sunlight, flushes all your body organs and brain, with oxygenated blood. This seems sensible as it refreshes your whole body and can naturally give an enormous lift in mood and general outlook. I do understand that this is not always easy to do because of the demands of parenthood and the nature of postnatal depression, but it is worth keeping in mind.

Summary

There are all sorts of situations that can get in the way of a smooth sailing breastfeeding journey. In this chapter, I have touched on the ones that are most common and that cause the most angst. It seems that by understanding and overcoming any difficulty, however slight, there is a significant degree of satisfaction and with it, an increase in knowledge and confidence.

If you have difficulties of any sort, it is worth working through them, using whatever help feels right for you. And remember that all the time, your baby is growing and changing. No sooner are you in one pattern of feeding and sleeping, then subtle changes take place, and you find your family rhythm changes.

Many parents will never encounter any of these *humps* in their breastfeeding journeys. I hope that in time this will be much more so, leading to longer, happier breastfeeding experiences than the present world breastfeeding statistics indicate.

Chapter 8

Complex challenges

No matter how things turn out, as long as a mother continues to give her child any human milk at all, it will be well worth the effort. Every drop of human milk is a precious, enduring treasure for a child, and feeding him at the breast even if there is no milk at all will be deeply satisfying.—Diana West, *Defining Your Own Success. Breastfeeding After Breast Reduction Surgery*, La Leche League International, 2001

The previous chapter encapsulated the most common situations that cause parents concern. All, with understanding and support, can be managed so breastfeeding can be continued and enjoyed.

The following situations are rarer—but the same applies. With information, understanding, the right kind of help and sometimes great patience, any challenging situation can be overcome. Although less common, they are important to discuss. If any of these situations concern you, this knowledge will help build confidence for you and those around you to seek support for your particular needs. The right support usually means people who really listen to what you are saying, and have the professional knowledge to understand and give appropriate suggestions for action. These are circumstances where an IBCLC can be very helpful to clarify, suggest strategies and refer on to specialised health professionals if necessary.

An IBCLC is trained in all aspects of breastfeeding and lactation. She (or he) can work with you through difficulties and is aware of the emotional and psychological impact that breastfeeding issues can have. Lactation consultants often work in hospitals, doctor's surgeries and private practice. Unless you have contact details of a local lactation consultant in your handy resource list, the easiest way to connect with one near to you may be by Googling: find a lactation consultant—or 'FALC' on the International Lactation Consultant Association (ILCA) Website.

Can you breastfeed after breast reduction or breast augmentation surgery?

Many women, for different reasons, have breast modification surgery during their pre-baby years. It may be a *breast reduction* to reduce the size of very large breasts. Surgery can relieve back and shoulder pain, improve posture and self-image. Or, it can be surgery to increase size, which is *breast augmentation*. Both types of surgery are common in some countries. They are often carried out at a time when the thought of having babies and breastfeeding is not considered. The surgeon may not even have been asked *−Will I be able to breastfeed?*

The most important aspect relating to breastfeeding after surgery is that you do want to breastfeed and are willing to *go the extra mile* to get the most positive outcome. Breastfeeding experiences for women who have had surgery often have different challenges than those who have not. Each mother's journey will be unique. Some will be able to breastfeed exclusively, while others will breastfeed successfully with supplementation.

It is helpful to make enquiries before your baby is born to clarify some aspects of the surgery. This knowledge will give you more indication of a realistic outcome. Useful information would be:

- The type of surgery and how was it performed. This is because some techniques keep more lactation tissue, nerves and milk ducts than others. When multiple milk ducts and nerves are severed or disrupted, there will be a lower milk supply.

- What the surgeon said about breastfeeding. Many will say, if asked, that breastfeeding is possible, but there is no guarantee.

- The length of time between surgery and pregnancy. The longer, the better because over time nerves and ducts will very slowly regrow. This is called *reinnervation* and *recanalisation*. This is helped by the monthly hormonal cycles for menstruation by stimulating breast gland and tissue growth.

- You may also choose to contact a lactation consultant who can help with suggestions to optimise milk production and assess the progress you and baby are making along the way.

When baby is born, follow the strategies for a great start to breastfeeding as suggested in Chapter 2. Skin-to-skin contact and early attachment for feeding will significantly help you achieve the best outcome.

Be as patient and persistent as you can. It is valuable to have close follow up in the first few weeks so that signs of adequate milk intake can be observed. For example:

- Is colostrum coming through with the initial early feeds?

- Is the let-down reflex working? Only some women feel this.

Others may feel *after-pains* (These are good signs if observed, as they indicate that the oxytocin hormone has been stimulated by baby suckling.)

- Is baby getting enough?

- Is baby starting to gain weight within normal limits?

If it appears that with proper attachment and frequent suckling, baby is unsettled and not gaining weight, strategies for extra supplementation that are appropriate for a breastfeeding mother can be discussed. These may be the use of medications called *galactagogues* to help production. A commonly prescribed one is called Domperidone. A supply-line with formula or donated breastmilk is useful as baby gets the needed additional milk, while suckling at the breast. Suckling stimulates your milk production. This can also be offered by the finger feeding method, a small cup, or by spoon. These strategies avoid baby having a silicon teat in his mouth, which can cause him to be less keen to attach and feed well at the breast.

Many women do breastfeed after breast surgery—a great resource that I recommend is Defining Your Own Success. Breastfeeding After Reduction Surgery by Diana West. (West, 2001)

Insufficient glandular tissue, or hypoplasia

I include this because of it being one of the less obvious situations that can cause breastfeeding difficulty. There are signs of hypoplasia that can be seen during pregnancy, but often they are not noticed or diagnosed. It can cause great distress for a mother with a new baby when she is following all the suggested tactics to get breastfeeding off to a good start, and not enough milk is being produced to satisfy her baby and maintain a weight gain.

While all breasts, big or small are usually ideal for breastfeeding, on rare occasions there are some that do not have enough of the actual milk making glandular tissue to produce a full milk supply.

The signs or *red flags* for this that could be noticed during pregnancy are:

- Breasts widely spaced apart - more than four cms. (Mohrbacher, 2012)
- Little or no breast changes during pregnancy
- Very unevenly shaped breasts
- Tubular, or cone-shaped breasts—sometimes with *bulbous* nipple area.

Breast hypoplasia does not mean that a mother can't breastfeed—it just means that she may not be able to produce all the milk her baby needs. Feeding as early as possible after birth, optimal attachment and frequent feeds will help with the best milk production. If extra milk is eventually required, it can be given by strategies as above, so that maximum breastmilk making stimulation is encouraged.

Special breastfeeding situations—breastmilk for all babies

It would be ideal for all babies to receive the parent/infant bonding benefits of feeding at the breast and the unique qualities of breastmilk.

> *A book by Alyssa Schnell called Breastfeeding Without Birthing is most informative, as it explains in detail the more unusual circumstances where breastfeeding will be an enormous help to the bonding and satisfaction of parents and infants.* (Schnell, 2013)

There are many situations where young, and even older babies are introduced into a family. Some by surrogacy, some by adoption, some into a gay or lesbian family. These infants can have the intimate connection of breastmilk and a breastfeeding relationship, in many different ways. This may be enlightening news to the many lesbian, gay, bisexual, transgender, queer (LGBTQ) people in relationships, who sincerely desire to have children to love and nurture. It may mean that a non-birthing parent in a same-sex relationship can induce lactation to breastfeed as well as the birthing parent. In these situations, breastfeeding is not easy to establish but with much thought, dedication, patience and persistence it is definitely possible. It also will open up easy options for gay couples to benefit from the bonding relationship with their infant by feeding skin-to-skin, not actually breastfeeding, but feeding at the chest. It may be that they have access to breastmilk from a reliable source. These parents need support and encouragement from like-minded people, family, friends and knowledgeable health professionals.

Induced lactation

Inducing lactation, sometimes called *adoptive lactation*, is the progressive stimulation of breasts towards milk production. It usually relies on prescribed hormone medication that imitates what your body would produce naturally if pregnant. The hormones are changed appropriately to mimic what happens at the time of birth, to start the production of milk. Along with this, a galactagogue (usually Domperidone) is prescribed to stimulate milk production further. Breast expression is encouraged giving milk-making structures in the body a message to make more milk to replace what is taken. (Newman and Pitman, 2006).

To assist in the continuation of milk production, frequent suckling between ten and twelve times a day is ideal. The reason for this is to encourage maximum stimulation for breast glandular tissue growth, as would happen in pregnancy. Avoiding dummies or pacifiers, keeping all suckling at the breast, also helps. If extra milk is needed, it can be given using a supply-line.

Several protocols may be used to promote lactation for feeding and nurturing a new or adopted infant. (Schnell, 2013 and Mohrbacher, 2012). There are also many strategies to encourage your baby or infant to learn to attach and suckle.

The success of induced lactation depends on the parent's goals. Part or all of a baby's milk requirements may be met. Some parents consider the more significant benefit to be the nurturing and bonding that occurs with their infant during skin-to-skin breastfeeding or suckling for comfort.

It is important to remember that breastfeeding is more than just about the nutrition—there are many other physical and emotional advantages from the closeness of breastfeeding. Any amount of breastfeeding is worthwhile.

Parents or future parents using an induced lactation protocol ideally need to work with the support of a physician who can finely tune the necessary hormonal medications or the particular plan you wish to follow. A lactation consultant who is familiar with the routine will be supportive physically and emotionally as the infant learns to attach, suckle and feed frequently enough to encourage continuous milk supply. A lactation consultant can also assess the infant's physical and developmental progress, and suggest strategies for extra milk intake if necessary.

Breastfeeding more than one –multiple births

In recent years there has been a marked increase in the birth of twins and triplets. A family history of multiple births may well result in more than one baby being born, but the advancement of fertility treatments for women who have delayed pregnancy until over the age of thirty has also had an impact on this increase. (Riordan and Wambach, 2009)

It can be overwhelmingly wonderful, amazing and joyful, but also absolutely daunting, to be confronted with the news that you are pregnant with twins or triplets. The thoughts that rush through your head may be: How will I cope? How will I feed? Will I have enough milk? The good thing is that usually you do have some time to acclimatise yourself with the idea and can gradually make plans for the birth and breastfeeding. A review of the *after birth feeding plan* in Chapter 2 will remind you of ways to help your babies have a positive breastfeeding start.

Knowing how breastfeeding works, assists you to understand that it is absolutely possible to produce enough milk for multiple babies. This knowledge gives you confidence in the fact that your milk supply depends on babies feeding—the more they feed, the more milk you will make. Whether you have two, three or more babies, your milk-making hormones will be stimulated to match what is needed. Your body is amazing.

Planning can help. Plan to breastfeed. If you are expecting multiples, be ready to adapt your *after birth feeding plan* to suit your particular situation. Let those assisting you with the births know that you plan to breastfeed and discuss how this can best be achieved under your circumstances. Do be prepared to be flexible and realistic, as with any births multiple or not, there are elements of unknown. If at all possible, you will have the support and encouragement of experienced midwives who are familiar with breastfeeding strategies for twins and triplets. (K, Gromada 2007)

- Have supports in place for when you go home because you may need to concentrate just on feeding and getting as much rest as possible in the first weeks and months. Grandparents, friends and family will all want to help, so when asked, suggest what might be truly helpful. Useful ideas may be making meals, cleaning, washing, ironing, shopping, or caring for older children. Ideally, helpers will be supportive and encouraging for you to breastfeeding the babies.

- Learn as much as you can about the expression of colostrum and breastmilk as sometimes babies are born early and may not be able to go straight to your breast for feeding. Your milk has specific protective advantages over manufactured milk, so it is great if you can avoid formula. This may mean frequent expression of colostrum and milk in the early post-birth stages, so being familiar with both hand and pump expression techniques will be helpful.

- Enquire about breast pumps—single and double, how they work, and whether the hospital has a supply that you could use if needed. Can you buy or hire one for use at home?

- Think about how you can make a comfortable *feeding nest* in your home with everything you might need while nursing—a comfortable seat, a special pillow, a place to put your drink bottle and snack, your phone, TV remote or a book to read.

- Learn about different feeding positions to try. Have contact with a multiple birth group by requesting information in your local area. You will be amazed at the helpful and supportive ideas that can be shared.

When babies are born.

- Ask to have them placed skin-to-skin on your (and perhaps your partner's) chests as soon as possible. Encourage their feeding within one to one and a half hours, or as soon as they initiate feeding cues. Even if the babies don't initially attach and suckle, the skin-to-skin will be an advantage for your connection with them as well as for future attempts at feeding.

- Initiate expression of colostrum if necessary, which may be the case if babies are born early, do not initially feed well, or if you or babies are unwell after the birth.

- In early days, observe and notice how each baby feeds—they usually will have their individual style and subtle differences.

144

- Ideally, each baby should feed eight to ten times in twenty-four hours.

- Have a chart for each one to keep ahead of who feeds when and on which breast. This may include keeping tabs on bowel actions and wet nappies.

- If any baby is not attaching well, get help from an experienced midwife or lactation consultant as early as possible.

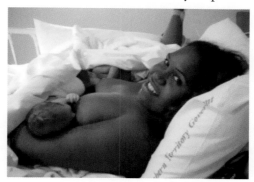

Babies that are born prematurely

It is not so easy to adapt your *after birth feeding plan* if baby or babies are born well before their due date, as there are particular challenges that parents and babies face. These depend on just how premature baby or babies are. Regardless, there is a far higher degree of dependence upon the specialised skills of medical and maternity staff to guide you through this often stressful time.

Your breastmilk is of great importance to any baby born early because it is designed precisely to match what your baby needs for his stage of development. Your pre-term milk changes according to your baby's growth.

Some of its unique qualities are:

- It has higher levels of protein, sodium, nitrogen, and magnesium, as well as increased concentrations of anti-microbial agents and immunological factors

- It is gentler on baby's kidneys

- It encourages baby's intestine to mature

- It is of great benefit to the growth of baby's immature brain

- It contains necessary ingredients like iron and zinc that are absorbed best from breastmilk

- It reduces the chance of infection

The important message for parents of premature babies is this: although daunting, breastfeeding is definitely possible and, with appropriate care, even very early babies ultimately do very well. The highly skilled staff caring for you and your baby or babies will guide you through the steps needed to initiate breastfeeding wherever possible. A significant part of this is supporting you to express colostrum, starting as early as possible after baby's birth. Despite the expert help, this may not be easy because of all your feelings and emotions connected with having baby or babies earlier than expected. However, having information about your colostrum, and knowing about breastfeeding in general, gives great incentive to enable you the best possible start. With patience and persistence, you can progress to exclusive breastfeeding, or work towards your personal breastfeeding goals.

Sometimes baby can go straight to your breast as in your *after birth feeding plan*, but this depends on his size, the degree of prematurity and physical condition. Each baby is different, and his feeding plan will be developed accordingly. That may include a tiny tube feeding directly into his stomach or small intestine until he is a little older and more mature. Again, as in the *after birth feeding plan* you can, wherever possible, have baby or babies held against your bare skin. This is sometimes referred to as *kangaroo care*. You and baby will benefit from this, providing that he is mature enough and depending on his particular circumstances. Staff generally know the value of baby's close contact with parents' warmth, heartbeat, and smell, and will be able to guide you as to when and how to do this safely.

As baby matures and progresses, your feeding plans will change, and often mothers become proficient at expressing their milk, even producing up to 50 per cent more than their baby needs. As already mentioned, expressing is important and should start as soon as possible after baby is born. An early established milk supply is helpful as baby transitions from tube or another feeding method, to feeding straight from the breast.

Summary

There are so many different scenarios because every mother and baby is unique. With some of the situations in this chapter, specific help and support are necessary for parents to attain their breastfeeding goals. Sometimes it needs to be ongoing for varying amounts of time, requiring parents to be patient, persistent and utterly determined. The information you have accrued will help you to be confident and reasonably assertive to receive the consistent support that fits in with your needs. No amount of time and effort put towards achieving your breastfeeding goals is wasted. Overcoming challenges, or even partly overcoming challenges can be rewarding, knowing that you have done, or are doing your best. Your baby will benefit from every bit of breastmilk received. He will also benefit from the love and closeness he has with you as you work through any of these challenges.

Chapter 9

Foods other than breastmilk—starting solids
How and when?

Eating should be pleasurable for everyone—adults and babies alike. Playing an active part in mealtimes and being in control of what we eat, how much to eat and how fast to eat it make eating more enjoyable. Early experiences of happy, stress-free mealtimes are more likely to give a child a healthy attitude to food for life.—Gill Rapley and Tracey Murkett, *Baby-led Weaning. Helping your Baby to Love Good Food,* Ebury Publishing, 2008.

This chapter is included because *when to start solids* is a common question among parents and has the potential to cause angst in the first year. It can be confusing. Over the years, there have been conflicting recommendations. Parents wonder how the breastfeeding part of nutrition fits in with the introduction of solids. In this chapter the how, when and why are explained. Strategies are suggested to make a natural, enjoyable and gradual transition that is harmonious with breastfeeding. Now that much more is known about babies' immune and digestive systems and the absolute value of breastmilk, all the major health authorities agree that there is no need to start offering other foods until around six months of age. Breastmilk or formula is the complete food until then. Despite this, parents are still bombarded with mixed information from food company advertising and different messages in the community, so it is no wonder there is confusion. Many myths abound, stemming from a lack of up-to-date information.

Why around six months?

This is when, developmentally, babies are usually ready to start experimenting with solid food. Before six month's of age, a baby's gut is designed to process only breastmilk efficiently. There is a higher risk of infections and developing allergies if other foods are introduced earlier. That is because baby's digestive and immune systems are immature and will let foreign proteins pass into their bodies easily, increasing the risk of sensitisation.

If you have a family history of allergies, it is wise to be cautious—even after six months, when introducing offending foods. Common foods that cause allergies include dairy foods, eggs, shellfish, nuts and wheat. If you are in this situation, discuss starting solids with a health professional. However, by breastfeeding exclusively for six months before introducing other food, you are reducing your baby's risk of developing a food allergy.

Overview of feeding

Babies, when in the womb, feed continuously, drinking and swallowing the amniotic fluid around them. In doing so, they get small tastes of the foods you eat that filter through. This is the start of the development of taste. After he is born, he will again be looking for frequent small feeds and is familiar with your smell and dietary choices. He may start his very first feed, attaching to your breast to suckle using natural feeding instincts and abilities. This is often called *baby-led attachment*. Baby, even at this early stage, has an element of control.

When he is *fed on demand* in the early weeks, he may have between eight and twelve feeds within twenty-four hours, continuing until his stomach and coping abilities change and develop to space out feeds a little. Every mother and baby gradually acquire their own feeding pattern. Baby self-regulates or controls his intake, taking only what he needs. According to ultrasound studies, his tummy empties in about thirty-five minutes. Breasts fill up in about the same time, which reinforces the fact that it is normal for babies to have frequent feeds.

Dr Howard Chilton, an expert neonatologist, says that when baby is suckling and swallowing, he is reminded of the bliss of the womb. Additionally, along with the breastmilk, comforting, calming hormones are released into his circulation. (Chilton, 2013)

Healthy eating becomes more established as baby grows with breastmilk. It continues to be the main source of nutrition in the first twelve months of life. It is the perfect fully balanced food, the quality of which stays the same for as long as baby breastfeeds. The additional introduction of family foods from the age of approximately six months to complement breastmilk is important in the progression towards a healthy eating pattern and proper nutrition.

If baby is given, for example, pureed food regularly in the early months, he will be less hungry for breastmilk, and so less breastmilk is produced because there is less demand for it. So, the premature introduction of solid foods can interfere with his main source of nutrition.

One of the disadvantages to the common practice of feeding babies pureed or mashed food via a spoon is that we are partly taking away the control they had with just breastfeeding, often encouraging them to eat more than they need. A caregiver might say, *just one more mouthful! Let's finish this yummy custard I have made you.* So already at this young age we can take away baby's ability to self-regulate by encouraging him to have more. In this way learning opportunities may be reduced. It may increase chances of not stopping when they have had enough later in life.

Additionally, the early introduction of solid foods may be related to excessive weight gain.

According to the World Health Organisation, 2017 statistics:

World obesity has tripled between 1975 and 2016

Currently, 39 percent of adults aged over 18 were overweight or obese.

41 million children under the age of five were overweight or obese in 2016

Obesity is a problem because it affects general health into adulthood. Because obesity in children around the world has become epidemic, children are developing obesity-related disorders that had typically been diseases of adults.

One of the great advantages of breastfeeding that is not often acknowledged is that it gives baby early practice in controlling his own appetite. When babies breastfeed, they stop when they have had enough. This is thought to be partly due to specific hormones in breastmilk. (Savino et al., 2009). It is impossible to force a baby to feed at the breast. The amount consumed at each feed varies according to what they need and how hungry they are. Consequently, breastfed babies are rarely overweight. They learn to stop when they are satisfied. They may well be avoiding obesity later in life.

How other foods can be introduced

Meal times should be happy times when family members can listen and learn from each other—even from a very young age. It is a social time, a time of inclusion. For baby, family meals are a broadening of the more personal time he spends with his mother as he breastfeeds. Babies generally show great interest in watching and imitating family activities from the age of four months. At that age, he may be interested in looking and touching and even mouthing family food but not eating, chewing or swallowing it. By around six months he will take a more definite interest in other food. This is because, developmentally, babies are sitting or nearly sitting up by themselves, and becoming smarter at reaching out for objects to put in their mouths. They love watching parents and siblings eat, and want to copy. They seem to enjoy handling food as much as experimenting with it in their mouths. As they do this, they are giving their mouth, lips and tongue good exercise that, incidentally, is a useful practice in learning to speak. Having this opportunity helps them eventually become more experienced in chewing and swallowing and, most importantly, having control over their eating process.

Babies do not need always to have special food prepared, pureed, and fed to them on a spoon. It can be beneficial to continue to let them take the lead as to what they eat, how they eat and how much they eat. Just as they do when breastfeeding.

When babies handle their food initially, it has little to do with hunger. It has more to do with curiosity and following what others do. They enjoy the feel of soft finger food and the attempts at manipulating it in their hands and mouth.

Foods which are ideal to start with between six and nine months are:

- steamed or lightly boiled vegetable pieces such as pumpkin, potato, broccoli, whole beans, or sugar snap peas.

- Fruit such as avocado, watermelon, banana and orange.

- Meat such as strips of warm lean beef, pork, lamb or chicken.

- Fingers of cheese, or savoury toast.

Cut foods into the size and shape that baby can handle easily; they learn themselves where to place it in their mouths and how to manipulate it so as not to gag or choke. They may gag as they experiment, but with practice, they will quickly become more adept at moving food into and around their mouths. They have the opportunity to learn about tastes, different textures, smells and have control as to whether they progress to chewing and swallowing or letting the food fall out. Just feeling new foods in their mouths must be an explosion of sensory stimulation for them.

What about the breastfeeds when baby starts solids?

Keeping in mind that when baby is first introduced to solid food, he is using the experience not necessarily for nutrition or calories, but for the colour, taste, texture, smell and sensuality of mouthing interesting things. So breastfeeds should at first continue with little change. He has a wonderful time practising his hand, eye and mouth coordination. Initially, it isn't something that will *take his hunger away*. Gradually, and usually over several months, baby becomes more adept at actually chewing and swallowing food, realising that it makes his tummy feel good; it satisfies part of his hunger. Often, around nine months of age his milk feeds reduce, and solid foods become more important to him. As with all stages of development, babies will vary as to how they progress with solid food and the reduction of milk feeds. Some move very quickly to a wide variety of foods, some thoughtfully and slowly. Usually, by around twelve months, babies have become adept at eating a range of family foods at main meal times, often with a small healthy snack in between. Some have even become quite clever at handling a spoon or other feeding utensil. Water in an open cup is a good way to introduce *other fluid* and can be offered at meal times. Providing baby can have a breastfeed when he needs, breastmilk will quench his thirst, and other fluids are not necessary. Offering water at mealtimes, however, will give him the opportunity to learn gradually that water does relieve thirst. It is not a good idea to give juice or other sweet drinks to babies, toddlers, or children. They can be addictive, and the high sugar content can damage their teeth.

So there is no need to consider *dropping a breastfeed* because baby has started solids. Continue to follow your baby's lead. He will let you know by taking less at breastfeeding times, or simply not want one or two of his usual breastfeeds because his body has adjusted to being satisfied by taking other foods. In the earlier months when starting solids, it is a good idea to encourage your lactation, or your continued milk production, by generally offering breastfeeds first, before the solid meals. This is so baby's appetite is not dulled because of a full tummy, making him less interested in his breastfeed. Less interest means less demand, and therefore less milk made. You may not want this to happen.

As time goes on, and baby is nearing the latter part of his first year, this may change. Solid food will probably become more important, and breastfeeds, although very valuable, may be less frequent, or accessed for comfort and closeness, rather than purely for nutrition.

Biting

I have heard many mothers say that they will stop breastfeeding when their baby gets teeth—the fear of baby chomping down on their sensitive nipples is just too much. In my experience, baby may occasionally do this, but it is rarely a problem if handled in the right way.

From approximately five months onwards your baby may be feeling irritation and discomfort in his gums as teeth start to push through. Occasionally during this time of teething, and usually at the beginning of a feed when he is waiting for a *let down* or at the end of a feed when he is sleepy, or just playing, he may give you a nip, which could make you startle and yelp. It is unlikely that he will do this when he is busy feeding actively because his tongue is over his lower gums and teeth when he feeds.

As with any undesirable behaviour in babies, or children, it is best to give as little reaction and attention as possible. If biting occurs, understand that your baby didn't plan to hurt you and that his gums are probably annoying him. Calmly say 'no' and bring him in closer to you as you try to continue the feed. If it happens again, firmly finish the feed by putting your finger into the side of his mouth to remove him from your breast. He will quickly learn that you mean business and that it is not acceptable for him to do this. Other useful strategies are to push down firmly on his gums using your clean finger before he feeds. This eases the pressure of the teeth pushing on gums and reduces the feeling of irritation when he feeds. At other times a cold teething ring can be soothing and encourage his teeth to cut.

Summary

In summary, the introduction of food other than breastmilk is an area to think and read more about. Different cultures have alternate ideas, and as already mentioned, there can be confusing messages from food company advertising. In my experience, parents, particularly first time parents, are often keen to move their baby into eating solid food before six months. There is no need to do so; it is too early and unnecessary. It starts the weaning process and alters the amount of breastmilk made. Of course, there are some exceptions, and it is always to be remembered that every mother and baby are uniquely different, and there may be paediatric advice to follow. However, letting babies take the lead when they are developmentally ready, in what and how much they eat in a family meal setting, does have commonsense merit.

Chapter 10

Sleep, glorious sleep!

Sleep—or more accurately, the lack of sleep—can be one of the most challenging aspects of parenting during the first year or two of a baby's life. At a time when new parents should be enjoying the process of getting to know their baby, this lack of sleep leaves them doubting themselves.—William Sears, MD, 2000

Some parents never have any issues with how or when their baby sleeps. However, sleep, or lack of it, does deserve a chapter of its own because for many parents, it can play a huge part in how they feel day to day. This, of course, can have an impact on breastfeeding. Lack of sleep is almost to be expected in the beginning as parents adjust to caring for a new baby day and night. Occasionally tiredness can escalate and become extreme, with parents becoming stressed and exhausted because their baby wakes frequently, or will not settle for sleep. Some women say they ceased breastfeeding because of fatigue.

This chapter explains what is really happening developmentally for babies as they gradually grow—why they are sometimes difficult to settle—why sometimes they don't sleep for long—and why some babies frequently wake during the night. Safe settling and sleep strategies will help you confidently manage any difficulties.

In the first couple of months or so when baby is quite young, you expect to feed frequently during the day and night, with many brief sleep periods. Expectations change as baby grows older. As the weeks and months roll on, breastfeeds usually become a little more spaced apart—most of the time, anyway. Often you find that there is one more extended stretch of sleep that develops somewhere in a twenty-four hour period. This longer sleep can be encouraged to be taken during the night rather than during the day by offering baby plenty of daytime feeds. If your baby seems to prefer a longer sleep in the day, you may choose to gently pick him up from his cot for a cuddle, cutting short this more extended stretch of sleep. Probably, soon after perhaps a nappy change and *talk*, he will show signs that he is ready for a breastfeed. Thus, you are encouraging more daytime activity and feeds, to help him *sort* his day and night rhythm.

To further encourage differentiation between day and night, have him sleeping in a well-lit room, where he can hear family daytime noises. In contrast, night time is darker and quieter, where you use less talking, singing, and stimulation. These strategies may help parents to have more uninterrupted sleep.

These suggestions are here to use if you choose. Babies will eventually get the gist of day/night rhythm without you doing anything.

When baby has a stretch of sleep between feeds of approximately five hours during the night, he is considered to have *slept through*, and this happens at different times for different babies. Some, when quite young, but many when they are well over five or six months.

Interestingly, as mentioned in Chapter 6, night feeds have advantages. As well as meeting needs for comfort and nourishment, they delay your menstrual cycle due to the natural suppression of hormones that stimulate ovulation. (Mohrbacher, 2012).

We all need our sleep, and because night feeds are part of the whole new baby package, it means that you need to make feeding at night as easy as possible for all concerned. Having baby's cot in your room is an ideal way to have baby close so that you can feed easily during the night, returning him to his bed when finished. In fact, maternity hospitals in some countries, the UK and Belgium for example, provide side-car cribs for newborns. These three-sided cots attach firmly to the mother's bed, allowing safe, close and easy access for breastfeeding. Mother and baby will often have a similar sleep rhythm and rouse from a deep sleep at the same time.

While no research has reported risks associated with side-car cots for infants, there are no studies on the safety of these devices in the home environment. Thus, there are no current mandatory safety standards at this time. However, research is underway, and recommendations may change in the future. (The ESCCaPE Trial, 2017).

Sleeping safety and SIDS (Sudden Infant Death Syndrome)

Sudden Infant Death Syndrome (SIDS) is the unexpected death of an infant under twelve months from an unknown cause. Globally, the rate of SIDS has declined because of the following safe sleep recommendations. (American Academy of Pediatrics, 2016)

• Always settle baby on his back to sleep and maintain this position throughout sleep

- Use a firm, flat mattress covered with a fitted sheet; no other bedding or soft items in the sleeping area

- Breastfeed to reduce risk

- Keep baby in your room close to your bed, but on a separate surface designed for babies

- Do not put soft objects, toys, crib bumpers or loose bedding in baby's sleep area

- Do not smoke during pregnancy and do not allow smoking around your baby

- Do not allow your baby to get too hot during sleep—dress him appropriately for the weather and environment

What about wrapping or swaddling?

Wrapping baby firmly and snugly can be an excellent calming, settling strategy for young babies—providing it is done safely. Important aspects to consider when wrapping are:

- Place baby on his back to sleep.

- Do not let baby overheat. Wrap according to the weather. For example, if it is hot and you are using a thin cotton sheet to wrap, baby would be dressed in a nappy only, or perhaps a nappy and singlet. If colder, he would wear a lightweight jumpsuit under the wrap.

Research suggests that while wrapping or swaddling can be useful, it is important not to let baby overheat. When too warm, he may go into a deeper sleep, making it more difficult to wake spontaneously, and therefore being at a higher risk of SIDS. He may also be less wakeful for breastfeeds, which may not be optimal for milk supply and weight gain, particularly in the early months. (Richardson, 2010)

- The wrap can be firm and snug around his body but loose around his hips allowing free movement and no tightness across his chest.

Some babies love to be wrapped—it makes them feel contained as if they were back in your womb. It also may give a sensation of what is coming next. Always put baby to bed on his back as statistically there is a much less chance of SIDS occurring. Sometimes, when the pattern of wrapping starts when very young, it continues as baby grows and is a regular part of the going to bed ritual. From about four months, when he reaches the age where he may roll, it is wise to wrap with his arms out or consider ceasing wrapping altogether.

The seven-week-old baby pictured likes to be wrapped for sleep. The following demonstrates a wrapping technique, leaving no tightness around his hip or chest areas. His hands are across his chest, and although contained in the wrap, they can move freely across his body because of the stretch in the thin material.

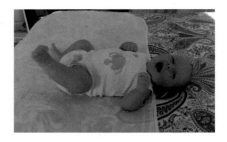

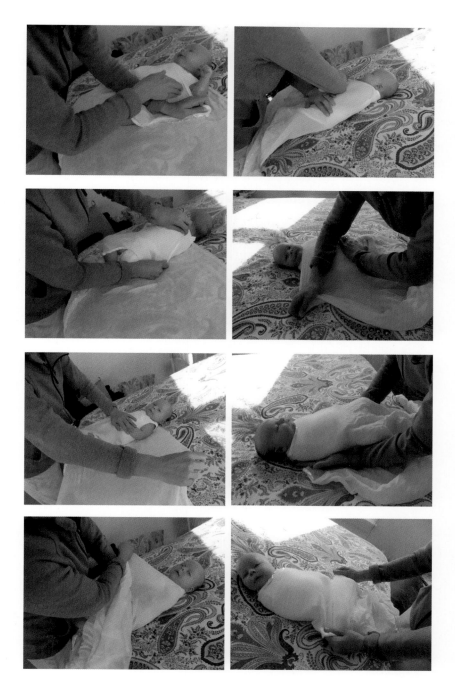

Progression—how sleep times change

Feeding and sleeping times are different for every mother and baby and evolve naturally. As baby grows, you will become more in tune with his particular feeding and sleeping pattern. Usually, babies do have some sleep between most feeds in the early months, but by about five months there will probably be a sleep time in the morning and another in the early afternoon, with a shorter nap in the late afternoon. There is much more awake time available for looking, listening, playing, talking and having fun.

By about seven months, many babies have dropped the late afternoon short nap, leaving just a morning and afternoon sleep. An example would commonly be sleeping from 9:30am to 11am and then from 1:30pm to 3pm. They are often tired and ready to settle for the night by about 7:30pm

By twelve months, many babies cope well with just one main sleep during the day and continue with an approximate 7:30pm bedtime.

This all sounds very streamlined and simple. It may be for some, but from my experience, not all babies settle well, and some frequently wake overnight for feeds or comfort.

What influences baby's sleep and what would we expect of babies in the first twelve months?

It is important to understand that it is normal for babies to wake during the night and is to be expected, especially in the first year of life. They wake for many reasons—often because of their normal sleep rhythm and as part of healthy development.

Baby's sleep rhythm

During a regular night's sleep, adults will drift into a lighter sleep approximately every two hours. When this happens, we might have a dream, sigh, or roll over, and we then return to deeper sleep. We are not particularly conscious of this happening.

Babies have sleep cycles similar to us, just a little shorter. They often go through periods when, instead of returning to sleep by themselves after a lighter part of their sleep cycle, they wake completely and need attention from parents. For example, they need a calming "Ssh...ssh...ssh" sound, a rhythmic pat, a cuddle, a nappy change and perhaps a breastfeed, before returning to sleep.

They need a degree of reassurance that a parent will come, or is there when they wake.

Normal development

When baby is around the age of about eight or nine months, some parents find that frequent night waking is a problem. It can even occur after months of having a reasonable night sleep pattern.

Around this time, frequent night waking is associated with baby learning to be separate from his parents. This is a normal part of development. Up until this time babies believe or think that they are joined to the main caregiver—which is usually the breastfeeding mother but can be any main person in baby's life. As their brain develops further, they register that they are separate from this person, and so start to go through a phase that is sometimes called *separation anxiety*.

You may observe this in other ways, for example, baby crying when he sees his mother walk out of the room. He thinks *I can't see her, so she's gone*, or *she's not coming back*. At this age, babies do not understand that she has only gone into another room and will be back shortly.

At this stage of development, babies may wake during the lighter part of their sleep cycle because of a niggling thought or concern about the absence of their special caregiver—it usually means *where are you*? They need reassurance that now they are more *separate*, their mother or main caregiver is near and will come when needed. The ones they love are all-important to them. Going to your baby when he wakes in the night is significant as it meets his fundamental needs to feel safe and secure. It helps him learn to trust, and that it is okay to be separate from you. Frequent night waking demonstrates that baby is going through this normal developmental stage. Additionally, it shows that he and his carers have a valuable attachment or bond that has already been enhanced by the closeness of breastfeeding. Of course, that is not to say that babies that don't frequently wake in the night are not firmly bonded with their caregivers. All babies are unique and build their relationships with those that love them in different ways.

Settling strategies for babies taking into account their age and development

Newborn and the first few months: Already mentioned are the ideas of wrapping, safe bedding and encouraging baby to differentiate between day and night.

Another strategy that many parents of very young babies have found useful during the day is to follow a pattern according to baby's needs. This requires you to tune into baby's signals, firstly for feeding, then into the signs that he is becoming tired. If he shows you, even very subtly, these tired signs and you put him to bed for sleep, he will be more likely to settle quickly. If these tired signs are overlooked and he becomes overtired, he will be more difficult to settle. This day pattern could be called a *feed, play, tired signs, sleep* pattern. This is how you can use it:

Feed your baby, both sides if possible. Often babies are quite sleepy and satisfied at the end of the feed. Instead of putting him straight to bed, try lying him down on a safe surface. He will probably become more alert, but still be very relaxed and happy. You may notice slow movement of arms and legs, open hands and a willingness to give you direct eye contact. This can be an excellent time for parents and siblings to have some playtime with baby. By play, I mean singing, touching, talking, smiling—most of all having direct eye contact with him. This is extremely useful for general development and enjoyment with your baby. After a short period—for a newborn it may be only ten minutes or less, you will notice some tired signs developing. The main four for a young baby are:

- jerkier movements of arms and legs

- hands more clenched than open

- facial grimace, or a head movement from side to side

- a little grizzle

When you notice his body language changing, if he is given a quick cuddle and put to bed even if he seems wide awake, he will probably settle fairly quickly and have a decent nap. If these signs are ignored, and he is further stimulated, he may be harder to settle for sleep. He has become overtired.

When you do put him into his bed, do so with a similar routine to help him get the feeling of what is expected of him. This might include a quiet cuddle, wrap, a few shhh, shhh's or a few pat pats. Every parent will develop their own words and routine when settling. Your baby will get the feeling of *Oh yes, I've had all my needs met—tummy full, cuddled, nappy changed and a lovely time with the ones I love. I am content and ready to sleep.* During the night when baby wakes, quiet feeds and putting baby straight back to bed usually works well. Leave the *play* for daytime only.

For older babies who are frequently waking during the night: It is normal for older babies to wake for some feeds. However, if they are around eight or nine months and are very frequently waking, it can become extremely tiring for parents. Babies around this age are most probably going through the separation anxiety stage of development as previously described, and are likely to wake for comfort and reassurance rather than because they are hungry. Regardless, when this happens night after night, and because baby is possibly getting a lovely breastfeed every time he wakes to help him go back to sleep, he continues in this pattern. It can become difficult to change. Although some night feeds are quite reasonable, a well-developed baby of nine or ten months does not need to be frequently fed during the night. Parents will often manage for a while with night wakings and feedings but, as tiredness mounts, it becomes too much, and at that point, it is often hard to get the specific help that is safe for you and baby.

What can you safely do about frequent night waking?

There are two main ways of handling frequent night waking with a baby under twelve months:

1. The first approach is what many parents do currently, and have done in the past. They continue to *go with the flow* and follow their babies' cues, feeding and comforting their baby no matter what age. These babies are fed without a second thought or concern. Many mothers view night feedings as an especially loved quiet time that they can have alone with their baby. They feed in a comfortable position, and little sleep is lost. These parents often do not have the extra pressures of returning to work or study and have partners who are relaxed about slight disturbances during their sleep time. Also, they possibly have the opportunity to have a rest or a *go slow* part of the day. They find that baby eventually stops waking of his own accord, except for the occasional feed. They haven't had to do anything different for this to happen.

2. The second is to discourage frequent night waking, by spacing breastfeeds to reasonable times during the night. To do this, you really need to take into account the whole twenty-four hour period—daytime as well as night-time. The most common helpful points to ask yourselves and consider are:

   • Does baby have regular sleep times during the day? Babies between six and twelve months generally need two daytime periods of sleep? A typical example would be 9:30am to 11am and 2:30 to 4pm. Daytime sleeps affect night time sleeping.

- Are daytime sleeps a reasonable length of about one or two hours long? It is best not to let baby sleep for too long, as they will be less likely to sleep at night. Gently waking baby after a moderate sleep is appropriate.

- Does baby have the opportunity to have plenty of active playtimes—on the floor, wherever you are and wherever it is safe? Babies settle and sleep much better when they are put into bed tired, but not over-tired.

- How does baby show you that he is tired? It is worth doing some *baby watching*, to consider the meaning of his noises and expressions. They are a big part of his growing communication skills.

- Do you go to baby in the night only when he really needs you? Sometimes babies will wake and talk or babble, or even have a tired grizzle and then return to sleep. Giving him a chance to do this and settle himself, may make a difference to the times you need to get up and attend to him.

- Is baby having plenty of breastfeeds during the day and, if appropriate, the opportunity for as much solid food as he indicates he wants at meal times? Babies sleep better if they are not hungry.

- Does baby have lots of close cuddling and talking during the day? This meets his need for physical and emotional contact with his loved ones? Babies sleep better when they feel *all is well.* His needs for touch and love are so important.

- Does baby have a calming bedtime ritual or a winding down time before bed? Babies respond well when they have a feeling of *what comes next* and a bedtime pattern can provide this.

- Is baby comfortable? He may be quite mobile in bed by this age, so a sleeping bag that is the correct size with a fitted neck, armholes or sleeves and no hood. Being warm, but not too warm is ideal. Babies sleep better when they have a regular bed arrangement that they feel familiar with.

- Do you put baby to bed when awake? Although this may not be what he is used to, it is being open and honest with him. Providing he is tired, and not overtired, he is more likely to learn to self-settle

- Do you use a specific bedtime or sleep time (day and night) language, encouraging others in the family to do the same? This helps babies to have a clear message of what is expected of them.

- Consider what is going on in the family. Babies often sense parents' stress, tension or disharmony. Parents' unease may be reflected in baby's behaviour. Employment changes, moving house or family separation can cause baby to have changes in sleeping habits.

Consider each of these points; some may make a significant difference in settling and sleep. Each time baby wakes with cries that are a definite *I need you,* attend to him in the same way. A brief cuddle and a few calming night-time words that reassure him may be all that is needed. If it is appropriate for a breastfeed, keep it quiet and brief. As breastfeeds are discouraged during the night baby will adjust by having a little more at different feeding times during the day.

For babies over twelve months: *Despite what you may have heard from websites, sleep experts, or even doctors—to leave baby to 'cry it out' as a means to solve sleep issues—is not a wise choice of management. This applies to any baby, regardless of age.*

As explained earlier, until baby is around six to nine months of age he would not understand the concept of being separate from you. To be ignored is like a dire emergency to him and very distressing. Consequently, his blood pressure rises, muscles tense and the stress hormone 'cortisol' floods his young brain. Babies who are left to cry unattended at night will likely be more clingy, fearful and fussy during the day. Putting in place an actual strategy for managing frequent night waking is really for babies who are twelve months or over. By that age, they are usually developmentally mature enough to cope quite well with parents taking a firmer stance without overwhelming them with stress.

It is not to be underestimated how hard emotionally, and physically, it can be for parents and baby to make changes. Baby is usually in a set pattern of waking and needing parents to resettle, often with a breastfeed. Parents sometimes suffer from extreme tiredness, which can be dangerous to their mental state and general health. Before considering making changes to night-time patterns, bear in mind the following points below, as well as those mentioned for younger babies.

- **Baby's age**: Is he at least twelve months old? Babies younger than this may not be developmentally mature enough to change night-time patterns. It is better to err on the side of caution by waiting until the baby is around twelve months so that when you do decide to make changes, you can do so with confidence.

- **Parents' expectations**: It is wise for parents to discuss with each other what they really need to achieve and why. Settling strategies and sleep changes are easier if parents work in unison, as consistency and persistence are essential. A steady relationship with proper channels of communication is important. When you do decide to make changes, don't be too impatient. It is best to be slow and consistent. Baby will need some persuading, especially if he has had lots of breastfeeds, or has been co-sleeping. Try to view this from your baby's perspective.

- **Baby's health**: Is baby healthy? This may mean a visit to your GP for a general check. It is not recommended to make changes when, for example, baby has an ear infection, a cold or anything else causing him to be unwell.

- **Baby's growth**: The doctor, midwife or Child and Family Health nurse can help you evaluate baby's growth by assessing his weight and length on the percentile charts in your health record book. If weight over time has been following an appropriate upward trend that approximately balances with his length, it will reassure you that baby is not waking because of hunger.

- **Have an appropriate daytime pattern for baby**: For some babies, this could mean two day sleeps and lots of active daytime play in between. Or he may have moved into a pattern of one longer day sleep. A typical example might be from about 12:30 after lunch to 3pm.

- Offer baby **plenty of food at meal times**, in addition to the usual breastfeeds. This gives you added confidence that he is not waking in the night because of hunger.

- During the day, give baby **extra hugs and cuddles** to help ease him into having less physical contact during the night.

- Babies love routines, so have **a consistent calming bedtime ritual** each time before his sleeps, so he knows what is expected and *what comes next*. This may be a quiet cuddle, a lullaby, reading a book together, or whatever you feel suits your situation- as long as it is a ritualistic, winding down time.

- **Separate feeding and sleeping:** If you have developed a habit of feeding baby off to sleep, it is helpful to change this by having a quiet activity between feeding and bedtime. An example would be a story or lullaby.

- **What else is happening?** Is this the right time for you as parents to make changes? For example, it may not be if your circumstances have changed or are changing—if you are moving house, if you have just started a new job or if there has been a separation or death. Do you have the energy right now?

- **Plan for encouraging a better night sleep pattern:** If you have decided it is necessary to make changes, it is a good idea to discuss your plan for change with a child health professional. Outside help can be a valuable tool in making changes, so check with appropriate people on your *resource list*.

If all of the above have been considered with adjustments made where necessary, your plan for change can be started with confidence. The following strategies will encourage less night-time waking:

1. Be honest with your baby. Tell him what you are going to do. For example, say, "Mum and Dad need more sleep, so if you wake in the night, one of us will come to help you go back to sleep, but without a breastfeed every time." Of course, baby won't fully comprehend, but he may well understand part of it and sense that his parents are being firm and fair and that they mean *business*.

2. Begin by putting baby to bed awake. Again, this is being open and honest and is helping him work towards self-settling.

3. Put baby into bed saying something reasonably minimal like: "night night, sleep time now, sweet dreams". Leave him if he appears to be settling, otherwise, note the noises he is making. If he is making grizzling, tired, winding down noises, you could continue to leave.

4. If baby begins making loud, distressed, crying noises when you go to leave the room, then stay with him. Give him a slow, firm pat about the rate of an adult heartbeat on the side of his body or chest, until he calms. When doing so, give him only minimal attention, perhaps just making

a ssh…ssh…ssh sound to go with your slow pat, pat. As he calms, or even goes to sleep, gradually slow the patting, remove your hand and leave the room. If he cries a little on your departure, this is normal. He is probably just winding down and will shortly go to sleep. If, however, the crying is distressed, recommence the patting and ssh-ing until he calms and you feel comfortable leaving the room.

5. If after 20 minutes, baby continues to cry with little change in urgency, despite your constant attention, pick him up and offer a drink of water from a cup. This will give him brief extra reassurance. But it is not very exciting for him—in fact not worth staying awake for! Put him back to bed and start again with the slow firm patting.

Whenever spending time settling your baby like this, ensure that your back is comfortable. A chair by the cot is a good idea.

6. When or if he wakes in the night, go to him and give reassurance with a brief cuddle. This may not be necessary every time he wakes. Then put him down saying the same words you used before—"night, night, sleep time now". Again, start the slow firm pats. This gives him the clear message that when he wakes in the night, the ones that he loves will come, but there are no great rewards for waking. He is having his main emotional and safety needs met and is being consistently reassured that you have not abandoned him. He may decide it is not worth waking up; it's actually more pleasant just to stay asleep. With consistency and perseverance, this course of action usually leads to a better night-time pattern and more sleep for parents.

7. Of course, if at any stage you feel it is appropriate to breastfeed your baby during the night, do not hesitate to follow your intuition. Many babies will continue to have a night time breastfeed with little sleep being lost—every mother and baby are different. There are no *rules*.

When does the night end?

Anytime after 6am is usually a reasonable time to start the day. If baby cries around this time, get him up. If however, he is still sleeping at 7:30am—even though you may have had a difficult night with him, and even though it might seem harsh, wake him and get him moving with his daytime pattern of feeds, playtime, and sleep. This will eventually have a positive effect on his night sleep.

The first few nights of using these strategies to encourage a better sleep rhythm can be particularly tiring for parents, who may already be feeling exhausted. If possible, start when you have minimal outside commitments and try to program some rest time into your day. If you can be consistent with using these ideas, reducing the number of night-time wakings (and feeds) will be possible. You will find that baby eventually gets *bored* with the same pattern happening repeatedly. As he is being reassured that you do always come when he wakes, he will naturally sleep better, only waking when he genuinely needs your attention or a breastfeed.

In my experience, taking the necessary precautions and following the above guidelines can be extremely helpful in encouraging better sleep habits and making family life happier and more relaxed.

Summary

There are many changes, particularly in the first year of your baby's life. Some are easy and delightful, and some are difficult and unexpected. Sleep, or lack of it, can make parents feel ground down to the point where the enjoyment of feeding, and parenting in general, is hampered. Having the resources to manage sleep concerns, if you choose, can make all the difference. Again, do not hesitate to source additional information and support to manage sleep or settling if you need. A professional outsider can often look at your *big picture* and suggest strategies that suit your particular situation.

Chapter 11

Returning to work—you can keep breastfeeding your baby if you choose

It is hard to be separate from your baby, but being able to nurse when you have reunited benefits both of you physically and emotionally. The look on your baby's face when you walk in the door after a long separation as he eagerly anticipates 'reconnecting' at the breast makes the effort of maintaining the nursing relationship well worth it.—Anne Smith *IBCLC, Breastfeeding Basics, 2015*

Returning to work is another step, albeit a big one, along the parenting journey. Continuing your breastfeeding relationship on commencement or recommencement of paid work has marvellous rewards, not only to you and your baby but also to the broader community. It demonstrates clearly that breastfeeding is highly valued and worthwhile. The more it is done, the more other mothers will do it too, and the more it will be seen as the norm. This chapter details how work outside the home while maintaining your breastfeeding relationship, can be efficiently managed.

In the past, many women felt that they had to wean before going back to work. Today, more women know their rights and are choosing to continue to breastfeed. They don't want to miss the benefits for themselves and their babies.

In most countries, there is an increasing number of women in the workforce, and many return to work well within twelve months after their baby's birth. The acknowledgement and acceptance of breastfeeding in the workplace has advanced over the past ten years, due to research demonstrating that everyone benefits when breastfeeding is encouraged and supported. Many organisations appreciate that supporting breastfeeding makes perfect business sense. It enhances their public image and reputation as being *family friendly*. Some have even been formally accredited as Breastfeeding Friendly Workplaces in Australia by the Australian Breastfeeding Association (ABA). Some other countries are way ahead of Australia regarding their support and facilitation of combining breastfeeding and work. It is wonderful to see progress in this important area.

These changes are significant because they mean that women indeed can return to paid work with confidence and expect to be supported and hopefully encouraged to continue breastfeeding their infant. The Sex Discrimination Act in 2011 strengthened these laws, protecting the rights of breastfeeding women.

Despite this, it is not easy contemplating and planning a return to work. You will be wondering how it will work for you, your baby and your employer. It all needs considerable thought. Some see it as a most significant obstacle following maternity leave. However, think of all the challenges already overcome since your baby's birth and what you have so far achieved. Going back, or entering the paid workforce while maintaining your breastfeeding relationship is another element in your parenting experience. It can be done.

One of the main keys to success and an important first step is to discuss your options with your employer, preferably while you are pregnant and before you start maternity leave. Investigate your workplace policies and if possible, talk to others who have combined breastfeeding and work. There may be aspects that could be improved upon for you and others in the future. You need to know what flexibility is available in your workplace. For example, is a gradual return to work a possibility? Are there opportunities to job-share or have flexible working hours? Could you work from home?

Employer benefits

There are definite benefits to your employer for having you back at work in a flexible arrangement. These might be used in discussion with your employer about your return to work. Some benefits are:

- As breastfed babies are protected in no small degree from illness and infection, mothers who are encouraged to maintain breastfeeding while in the paid workforce will have lower absenteeism to care for sick infants. This therefore leads to a steadier workflow and better productivity.

- Mothers who are supported in this parenting role will be likely to return to work sooner, be more committed and have positive employer/employee relationships.

- There is the very real likelihood of less staff turnover because skilled staff members are retained. Consequently, there are reduced costs in staff training and thus a higher financial return.

- All organisations benefit from having a *family friendly* public image. Today, more and more companies are adopting family-friendly work policies, which is commonsense regarding economic efficiency and the ability to retain skilled employees.

How to manage work and breastfeeding.

The situation is different for every mother, baby and family. However, review these strategies and use what is appropriate and feels right for you and, of course, see what works best.

Making the transition, while maintaining the feeding pattern you want, depends on many personal factors, such as baby's age, your distance from work, your child-care arrangements, your particular type of work and the support you have at home. Flexibility is essential because even though you may have had an appropriate discussion with your employer, your plans may change, and different ideas may evolve as you move towards your return to work.

As stated above, there needs to be considerable thought and planning into a move such as this—it involves separation from your baby, maintenance of milk supply and vital milk expression at work.

The elements to maintain milk supply that need negotiation, relate to breaks from your work to express. Usually, lunch, morning and afternoon tea times will be sufficient. You may need to discuss other times, depending on baby's age. Your requirements for this will be privacy where you can use an electric pump or hand express with freshly washed hands in comfort. You will also need somewhere to safely store your milk.

A general guide for lactation breaks in an eight hour day:

- For a baby under four months of age: 3 x 20 minute breaks

- For a baby who is six months of age: 2 x 20 minute breaks

- For a baby who is twelve months of age: may only need 1 x 20 minute break

Your main needs are:

- a private room, with a power point if you are using an electric pump

- a fridge

- a hand basin with running water

- a comfortable chair

Emotions play a large part in how you feel about this. Once baby is born and you have created a special bond with him, your reasons for returning to work may feel blurred and may need to be reassessed. Your head may say one thing and your heart may say another, which can be quite stressful. This is normal. Most mothers find the thought of being separated from their baby emotionally difficult, despite maintaining their breastfeeding connection.

Here are some tips that you may find useful:

- **Maintain contact with your employer.** Keep them informed about your plans or changes to what was discussed or negotiated. Their support and understanding of your situation make a difference as to how you feel about returning to work.

- **Consider the age of your baby**. Successfully combining paid work and breastfeeding is more difficult the younger a baby is. If baby is under six weeks, your milk supply may not be fully established, and your body may still be adjusting from being pregnant and giving birth. Feeding patterns are often irregular, and milk expression at work would probably need to be more frequent to maintain milk supply. There can be more flexibility for an older baby. From the approximate age of six months, when babies generally begin taking other fluids and solids, there is usually more of an established feeding pattern, and a reduced need for breastmilk. Not as much is required, and some daytime meals can be replaced with solids and water. For an even older baby, parents will often develop the pattern of breastfeeding before and after work, in the evenings and during the weekends.

- **Explore your alternatives** for work if you are in the position to be able to discuss possibilities with your employer. Attempt to reach an arrangement that suits you best. These may include:

  - Taking as much maternity leave as is feasible and is financially possible for you
  - A gradual transition back to work
  - Working from home for some or all of your work
  - Job sharing

- Having baby brought to you for some feeds, by a partner or carer
- Flexible starting and finishing hours around core work tasks
- Combining breastfeeding with some formula feeds
- Getting extra help in the home to reduce household tasks

- **Make arrangements for a carer** who is supportive of you breastfeeding your baby. This could even be before the baby is born, which may take the pressure off you when the time for your return to work draws near. Searching for the right person at the last minute can be stressful and takes time and energy. You may need to educate her or him regarding handling stored or frozen breastmilk and your ideas of a system for preparing and labelling bottles. You could choose to share information about breastfeeding, explaining that feeding is a time of closeness and social interaction and that you would like baby cuddled at feed times.

- **Become familiar and confident with expressing your milk** before returning to work. Practice expressing by hand (refer to Chapter 7) and consider hiring or buying an electric breast pump to experiment with. Everyone is different, but most mothers find a quality electric pump quick and efficient, with the advantage of being able to express both breasts at once if desired. There are several excellent pumps on the market, so it is worth researching what is available and which type suits your situation best. Becoming familiar with expressing will build confidence and possibly the bonus of a useful stock of expressed breastmilk to have on hand in your freezer. This can be very reassuring.

- Practice giving expressed milk to baby. Most babies, after milk supply and feeding patterns have been established, are happy to feed from a bottle with a teat. Occasionally this is not the case, and baby might refuse to accept the bottle. It may be helpful to have the carer who will be feeding your baby when you are at work, have practice feeding the expressed breastmilk before you commence your working routine. You may need to leave the room for baby to feel comfortable to drink from the bottle with his carer. This may be hard for you as a parent and, initially for the carer. But be reassured that if your baby is hungry enough when away from you, he will eventually take milk from a bottle. If baby is old enough, for example eight months and on, and is refusing to drink from a bottle, he may be able to drink from a small cup or through a straw. Ensure that your carer is confident feeding your baby, enabling you to be free to concentrate and enjoy your work as much as possible.

When you do begin work, expressing and storing breastmilk is vital for breastfeeding maintenance. If your milk is not expressed, you may have uncomfortable feelings of fullness, as well as risks of engorgement and possibly mastitis. Also, most significantly, your supply will reduce. The amount of milk you produce depends on regular, effective removal from your breasts, whether this is by baby suckling or by expression.

Successful breastmilk expression depends on how your milk *lets down*. This is usually so much easier when baby suckles at the breast and naturally stimulates the surrounding nerves to release oxytocin. This, in turn, causes the milk to be squeezed down towards the nipples and eject out as baby feeds.

Tips for comfortably expressing your milk

When expressing away from your baby, there are several strategies you can use to simulate baby suckling. Once you get into a pattern, it becomes easier and easier.

- Work towards having a ritual or routine for expressing—this helps the milk flow more quickly
- Try to have specific times that you express, for example tea and lunch breaks
- Ensure you are warm, comfortable and in a private setting
- Wash hands and have clean equipment ready
- Gently massage your breast in circular movements towards the nipple, spiralling around and then rolling your nipples between your fingers several times
- Stroke your breasts lightly from the top and bottom of your breasts, towards your nipples
- Shake your breasts gently while leaning forward, so that gravity helps milk to eject
- Focus your mind on your baby, think of your baby's smiles and talking noises; a photo or piece of their clothing may help
- Don't wait for breasts to become full before expressing, as fullness can signal the milk-making hormones that they need to slow down milk production. This is especially so if it happens frequently.

Leaking breasts

If at work and you feel the tingling of the beginning of a *let down*, (you may have been fondly thinking about your baby) pressing firmly on your nipples for several seconds can prevent leaking. This you can do by quietly folding your arms across your chest. Do consider that this tingling may be a message, suggesting it is time to express some milk.

In any situation where your feeding pattern changes, such as described above where you are expressing during the day when you were previously breastfeeding at these times, be aware of how your breasts feel. Observe your breasts for any patches of redness or soreness, as they may be early indicators of mastitis. This, however, is fairly rare when breastfeeding is well established, but it is worth mentioning because any progression can be averted with early action or intervention. For more information on mastitis, see Chapter 7.

Collection and storage of your breastmilk

Breastmilk storage bags can be purchased from most pharmacies and are useful for collection and storage of breastmilk, as are glass or BPA-free plastic bottles.

When buying any bottle for milk storage, check they do not contain the chemical bisphenol or BPA. This is used to harden plastics. There are concerns that this chemical may leech out into milk when heated, with possible harmful effects to infants. (Zuckerman, 2018).

As you collect your breastmilk at work, it needs to be placed in a fridge or an insulated bag or box containing a freezer pack. Once correctly refrigerated it will keep easily for days so you can have the option of having your caregiver use it the next day or, if frozen, anytime later. Batches of breastmilk expressed during a twenty-four-hour period can be chilled and then put in the same container and stored in a fridge or cold pack.

Freshly expressed breastmilk should be cooled in the fridge before being added to other chilled or frozen breastmilk. *Do not add warm breastmilk to frozen milk.* Expressed breastmilk may look bluish, yellowish or even brownish, and may separate with the creamier milk towards the top. This is normal and will mix quickly, given a gentle shake.

To thaw for use

To thaw frozen breastmilk, you can either hold the container under warm running water until heated to room temperature, or thaw slowly by placing in the fridge the day before it is to be used. Swirl gently to mix. Do not shake vigorously. It is not recommended to thaw or heat milk in a microwave because some of the important components can be damaged or destroyed, reducing its quality. Also, microwaves tend to heat unevenly which can result in *hot spots* of milk that could burn baby's mouth. Once breastmilk is thawed it should not be re-frozen, but can be kept in the fridge and used within twenty-four hours.

The following is a reference guide for storage of breastmilk—used with permission from Kelly Bonyata *kelly@kellymom.com* Updated February, 2018.

HUMAN MILK STORAGE - QUICK REFERENCE CARD		
	Temperature	Storage Time
Freshly expressed milk		
Warm room	80-90°F / 27-32°C	3-4 hours
Room temperature	61-79°F / 16-26°C	4-8 hours (ideal: 3-4 hours)
Insulated cooler / icepacks	59°F / 15°C	24 hours
Refrigerated Milk (Store at back, away from door)		
Refrigerator (fresh milk)	32-39°F / 0-4°C	3-8 days (ideal: 3 days)
Refrigerator (thawed milk)	32-39°F / 0-4°C	24 hours
Frozen Milk (Do not refreeze! Store at back, away from door/sides)		
Freezer compartment inside refrigerator (older-style)	Varies	2 weeks
Self-contained freezer unit of a refrigerator/freezer	<39°F / <4°C	6 months
Separate deep freeze	0°F / -18°C	12 months (ideal: 6 months)

These guidelines are for milk expressed for a full-term healthy baby. If baby is seriously ill and/or hospitalized, discuss storage guidelines with baby's doctor.

How much does baby need?

As discussed in Chapter 7, it is difficult to know how much baby needs each feed because there is such feed-to-feed variability. Also, estimating the approximate amount that your baby needs depends on factors such as his age and stage of development, whether he has solid food and other drinks, and how long you will be away from him. Generally, a rough guide for his feed amounts can be calculated by multiplying 180mls for each kilogram of body weight, and dividing by the average number of feeds in twenty-four hours.

I do say approximate needs because each baby will want different amounts, but you could start with this calculation and adjust the amount according to how much he drinks when away from you.

The calculation has been based on formula fed babies, so should be more than adequate for breastfed babies.

Examples of approximate amounts of milk for each feed:

A three-month-old baby weighing five kilograms and having eight feeds in twenty-four hours would need approximately 110 mls at each feed. *180 x 5 divided by 8.*

A six-month-old baby weighing seven kilograms and having six feeds in twenty-four hours would need approximately 210 mls. *180 x 7 divided by 6.*

Ideally, you can share all the relevant breastfeeding information with caregivers, so they work with you to make the transition to work and the continuation of breastfeeding as easy as possible. A useful tip would be for the carer to have a small amount of extra breastmilk on top of the calculated amount to take the edge off baby's hunger. If it is expected that you will soon return from work, a full feed would be inappropriate as it would dampen his enthusiasm for a breastfeed once connected with you.

This all may seem a lot to organise when considering your return to work and it is understandable that it may seem challenging. However, it can be viewed as another enriching step in the parenting process that can be managed with a little forethought and planning.

Maintaining your milk supply

- After a few weeks of juggling work and breastfeeding, you will be amazed at how your body and breasts adjust to making the right amount of milk for your baby

- During the day, squeeze in as many breastfeeds as you comfortably can. This could mean one in the early morning, even one at the caregiver's before you leave, a couple of evening breastfeeds and a before-bed breastfeed.

- Breastfeed full time whenever you are not at work. To maintain and build up your milk supply, it is good to have days when you frequently breastfeed to make up for the times when you and baby are separate. Don't give bottles when you could breastfeed. Pumping does not stimulate the breasts to produce milk as well as a nursing baby does. Breastfeeding when together ensures that baby stays interested in the breast.

- Many working mothers find that their supply dwindles towards the end of the week, but after nursing frequently over the week-end, their breasts feel much fuller for the start of the next working week.

- Often babies who are away from their mother during the day, slip into a pattern of feeding more overnight. They reverse their daily patterns by sleeping more and feeding less during the day. This is where having baby's cot close to the parental bed is handy as baby can be placed back into the cot after feeds with little sleep lost.

- Take care of yourself by considering ideas that may help to make it easier. The extra demands of managing your job and maintaining your breastfeeding relationship will take up most of your time. When you breastfeed, view it as your special time to rest and relax. Have nourishing snacks during the day, and when you first get home. Simplify life as much as possible by getting help if you can for household tasks like shopping, cooking, and cleaning. Try to share as many of the household tasks as you can and remember that giving your baby your milk is one of the best investments in your child's medical, emotional and intellectual future.

Other benefits for mothers, babies and families

- Continuing feeding with breastmilk decreases anxiety or grief about the separation from baby when returning to work. Breastfeeding your baby after a time away at work is a satisfying and relaxing way to reconnect. That special nurturing bond is maintained.

- Breastmilk is the perfect food, resulting in healthier babies, which means optimal opportunity for their speech, physical and mental development. Plus, less time and money spent on doctors visits and pharmacy costs because of illness.

- Breastfeeding is cheaper, and therefore of financial benefit to families.

- Already mentioned, there are long-term advantages for mother and baby that relate to the reduced risk of future health problems.

- The breastfeeding parent is able to maintain career momentum and enjoy the consequent advantages.

Advantages for the community and environment

- Because breastfeeding and breastmilk reduce the risk of illness and infection, the general community is healthier. It is like an investment in the future, as the long-term benefits include less risk of obesity, Type 2 diabetes, breast and ovarian cancer, heart disease and osteoporosis. All this has significant implications for community health and happiness, and results in a more robust workforce.

- Breastfeeding saves our health care systems millions of dollars each year.

The estimated health benefits of breastfeeding translate to reduced annual health care costs totalling 312 million dollars in the UK, $6 million in Brazil and $30.3 million in urban China. (The Lancet Breastfeeding Series. Key messages and Findings, 2016)

- Breastfeeding leaves no *footprint* and is, therefore, an asset to our environment. No dairy farms are needed for breastmilk; no energy is consumed to make it in factories, no resources are needed in packaging, no fuel is needed to transport breastmilk to shops and then to your home. There is no electricity or hot water needed to heat it, and it is time efficient as it can be given anytime, anywhere.

Throughout all of history, women have been creative about combining motherhood and work. All the reasons you chose breastfeeding are still important, and some are even more important now.—The Womanly Art of Breastfeeding, 8th *Edition, 2010*

Summary

Although it is not always easy maintaining a job and your breastfeeding relationship, remember the overall benefits. The period in your working life when feeding arrangements need to be made is very brief. As with all breastfeeding matters, there are no set rules and the strategies that you can use, or do not use, are mostly a matter of what works best for your family and work situation.

Chapter 12

Weaning

Ideally, the time for weaning is a joint decision in which both the mother and the baby reach a state of readiness to begin around the same time. However, this is not always the case. The child may be ready before his mother, or the more often, the mother is ready before her child.—Jan Riordan and Karen Wambach, *Breastfeeding and Human Lactation.* 4th Edition

Hopefully, you are now well settled in your baby feeding and nurturing journey. If there were any difficulties or hard times, you have overcome them. You are comfortable feeding anywhere, anytime, without a second thought. At some stage, you may start to wonder about weaning—just how it happens. This chapter explains the many weaning situations for parents with babies of differing ages and stages of development.

Weaning your baby from the breast can happen in many ways. It depends on your baby's age and stage of development, and the reasons for weaning. There is no recommended or ideal time, and weaning will occur differently for every individual mother and baby. It is immensely valuable, of course, to continue for at least twelve months as recommended by major health authorities and then for as long as you and your baby want after that. There is no set time that you *should* wean. In fact, the weaning process starts when you first introduce solid food and other fluids at about six months of age. It is a process. Your milk supply gradually adjusts to accommodate the increase in nutrition from other sources. Weaning ends when the last breastfeed is given.

You may notice when considering weaning, that particular feelings and emotions are aroused that can seem confusing. These can range from being very positive to those of anxiety and sadness. You may fluctuate between responses. This is very normal and understandable when you acknowledge that breastfeeding is far more than just a form of nutrition. It is a way of parenting, and it forms a deep relationship between mother and baby.

So when baby weans, even if planned, a mother can feel a sense of loss, like the grief experienced when any relationship goes through significant change. Emotions may be compounded by the natural shift in hormones as baby weans.

Prolactin is a hormone that is needed for milk production but also promotes feelings of wellbeing and calmness. Oxytocin, also known as the love hormone, is required for the let-down reflex when baby feeds.

As these hormones reduce when baby weans it is understandable that they have an impact on how you feel. The faster weaning takes place, the more these invisible body changes may be felt— sometimes as a temporary dip in emotional wellbeing. The slower, more gradual weaning allows hormones to readjust back to a normal pre-baby rhythm slowly. Many mothers are not aware of these changes.

Weaning can occur in several broad categories

- Rapid weaning
- Mother's choice to part or fully wean
- Natural weaning

Rapid weaning

Breastfeeding needing to cease as quickly as possible can be the most difficult type of weaning. It usually occurs for reasons beyond a mother's control, like a family crisis, or treatment for a medical condition needing medication that is incompatible with breastfeeding. Alternatively, it may be that the mother has simply chosen not to breastfeed any longer and wants to terminate quickly. However, emotional aspects for both mother and baby, as well as physical symptoms, need to be considered.

The closeness of breastfeeding is a comfort for baby. This can be replaced to some degree by extra hugs, cuddles and skin-to-skin contact with parents.

In these cases, weaning needs to be tailored to accommodate the specific situation and depends on the time mother has to wean. The slower baby is weaned, the better, with breastfeeding being replaced gradually with bottle feeds, unless baby is old enough to feed from a cup. If mother only has a few days to do this, she could alternate breastfeeds with bottle feeds on the first day, expressing just enough for comfort between feeds. Over the next days, the other feeds could be phased out, continuing to express a little milk when breasts become full or uncomfortable. Breasts will naturally and gradually stop producing milk if they are not receiving the stimulation of baby's suckling.

Nursing strike

Rarely and usually for no apparent reason, a baby who has been breastfeeding well will go on strike, refusing both breasts. This, of course, can be very distressing for the mother, as it can last for several days. Often baby is unhappy too. If baby is under twelve months, he has a physical need for breastmilk, so the strike is not because he naturally wants or needs to wean himself. It is more likely to be related to being unwell with an ear infection or a cold, or mouth pain due to teething, or thrush. It could also be caused by emotional factors, such as family disruption and loud noise. Or perhaps he has had a series of feeds given by bottle and is rejecting the change back to the breast.

If this occurs, consider going back to the basics of calm, skin-to-skin cuddling and offering a breastfeed before solid food. The laid-back position described in chapter 5 will enhance natural feeding behaviour, and encourage his instinct to attach and feed, in his own time. Protect your supply by expressing regularly, and if in any doubt about baby's health, see an appropriately qualified health professional.

Planned weaning—fully or partially

There are many reasons why a mother may wish to discontinue feeding. Whether fully or partially, weaning is best to be approached gradually, cutting down on one breastfeed per day every few days and replacing it with formula if baby is under twelve months of age. If baby is over twelve months, you may choose to go straight on to full cream cow's milk. This can be given via a cup.

It often suits mother and baby to maintain some breastfeeds, for example in the early morning and in the evening. This can be referred to as partial weaning, and these breastfeeds can be maintained for as long as you and your baby decide. Many women partially wean when they return to work, using some formula given by a carer during the day.

If feeding is to be via a bottle, think about which feed is least needed by your baby, or which feed is the least convenient for you to give. Many parents choose the late afternoon or evening one. It is sometimes helpful if someone other than mother gives baby the feed. Whether it is taken easily or with some resistance depends on whether baby is familiar with feeding from a bottle. Some babies will have had expressed breastmilk from a bottle.

After a few days, or longer, when baby has that bottle regularly, introduce another at the next time during the day that you think will work best. It may be the second feed of the day, for example. Continue in this new pattern for a few days, or even weeks, if that is what you decide. Continue reducing the breastfeeds and replacing them with bottles. This allows your milk supply to reduce slowly, avoiding discomfort and the risk of mastitis. If, during the process, your breasts do feel full and uncomfortable, express just enough to relieve the discomfort. If you have some stored expressed breastmilk in the deep freeze, this can be used before formula to avoid waste. If baby is over twelve months of age, milk drinks could include a small cup of cows milk as part of a mealtime pattern.

Extra hugs, cuddles and plenty of other food are helpful during the transition period, and your baby will gradually lose interest in feeding at the breast. Because solid food becomes a major source of nutrition after eight or nine months, it is a good idea to give the bottle of formula after meals—for example, before morning and afternoon sleeps and before bed at night. The amount will depend on the age of your baby and how much if any he is having in a cup at meal times. Your baby will usually let you know how much he requires by taking as much as he needs when it is offered.

If you are weaning an older baby, perhaps an active toddler, the following strategies can make it easier:

- Shorten the length of the breastfeed

- Delay breastfeeds, using distraction

- Feed with other food and drink before regular breastfeeding times, such as when baby wakes in the morning

- Have different daily routines

- Use a dummy for extra sucking

Weaning in this way takes varying amounts of time. However, it can be achieved quite quickly, even over a period of days, depending on baby's age and stage of development and your reasons for weaning. It can also be as comfortably gradual as you choose.

Generally, the time and process of weaning is negotiated between you and your baby and is a very personal decision. It certainly should not be influenced by social pressures, well-meaning friends, family, or anyone else in the community telling you when it should happen.

The benefits of breastfeeding remain as baby grows. Even though he may be receiving nutrition from solid meals and other fluids first introduced around six months of age, there are genuine advantages in continuing breastfeeding until you and your baby are ready to wean.

Some advantages of feeding an older baby

- Breastfeeding comforts a tired, upset or hurt toddler and gives both mother and infant some quiet, restful time together

- The hormones, as discussed, are relaxing

- Baby continues to have fewer episodes of illness because of the support to his immune system; the living cells in breastmilk deter infection

- Superior oral and possibly speech development because of the way the baby's face and jaw muscles are used

- Tandem feeding is possible if a new baby is born

If pregnancy occurs while you are breastfeeding, you and your older baby may be keen to continue during the pregnancy and when the new baby arrives. This is *tandem nursing*. Due to hormonal changes, breastmilk will taste slightly different, and this may encourage a natural wean situation. Other older babies or toddlers will continue, regardless of these changes. There can be some challenges during this time. Your nipples may become sensitive, and your milk supply decrease as it returns to more to colostrum-like milk in the later part of pregnancy. This is your body preparing for the birth of the new baby. Once the new baby is born, it is wise to let him have priority, establishing proper attachment and colostrum intake. Your older baby may have a renewed interest in breastfeeding, which can result in him initially having loose bowel actions from the laxative effect of colostrum. However, this extra nursing will ensure a copious milk supply for the new baby. When a mother is feeding both baby and toddler in this way, it is important that she eats and drinks well, and rests when she can.

Natural weaning

Natural weaning occurs when your child simply outgrows breastfeeding in his own individual way—when he takes more interest in other parts of life. Breastfeeding becomes less important to him. It is not usually a sudden decision—on the contrary, it is a gradual process, and your breastmilk supply diminishes slowly as he has less breastfeeds. You may go for a day here and there, without feeding, then two days, then three or more, until you realise that you and your baby have weaned naturally. You may not even remember the actual last time you breastfed. The transition is just another of your child's normal developmental steps. Sometimes babies will keep a preferred breastfeed, such as the early morning one, or just before bed, until that too becomes erratic, less frequent, and eventually ceases. This is a natural way to wean, with no ill-effects to mother or baby. When an infant is weaned in this way, your breasts will not be engorged or uncomfortable, and your hormones will adjust over time.

After weaning

As already mentioned, after weaning and, depending on baby's age and circumstances, there can occasionally be feelings of sadness and loss. This is related to the strong attachment that is not broken, but just changed. It is usually short-lived as other ways of comforting and nurturing are used successfully, and parents are faced with new and exciting stages of their baby's development.

Breastfeeding suppresses ovulation and therefore delays menstruation. This means that during the process of weaning, or at any time during your lactation, your monthly cycles will return. They may be irregular for a few months before they settle into their usual pattern. This also means that you will become fertile again and you may, or may not, consider contraception strategies.

Some women find that to prevent weight gain they need to cut back a little on their food intake. For others, this is not a concern. Again, it is an individual process.

After weaning, you may find that your breasts are soft and flat. However, they will gradually regain much of their pre-pregnancy firmness after several menstrual cycles. It is a myth that breastfeeding ruins breasts, as breast changes occur during pregnancy, whether you breastfeed or not. The area around your nipple, the areola, tends to remain darker than before pregnancy. If you happen to have stretch marks on your skin, these tend to fade gradually to faint white lines.

Some mothers experience breastmilk secretion for several months after they have ceased breastfeeding. This diminishes gradually until it is a colostrum-like consistency, and eventually stops. This is normal.

Summary

As stated, weaning can occur in a wide variety of ways. It happens differently for every mother and child according to the physical, emotional and practical needs in the family. Sometimes it evolves in a planned way, and sometimes as a natural milestone in a child's life. It starts when solids are first given and ends when your infant has his last breastfeed. The nutritional, emotional and general health benefits continue throughout breastfeeding and, of course, stand you and your baby in good stead for the years ahead.

Chapter 13

Resources and references

All's fine now, it is going well, and I love breastfeeding. I'm glad I persevered. I thought after eleven years in a professional environment, managing a variety of complex situations, this would be a breeze. I read books, listened to friends, attended every breastfeeding and parenting class that I could. But I found the first months hard. It is just so different from what I thought. What made a difference for me was asking questions, questions, questions. And nobody seemed to mind!—Susan Downfield quote, used with permission, *Parenting Class*, 2013

Breastfeeding is an instinctual and natural act, but it is also an art that is learned day by day. The reality is that almost all women can breastfeed, have enough milk for their babies and learn how to overcome problems both large and small. It is almost always simply a matter of practical knowledge and not a question of good luck.—La Leche League, 2018

It can be one of your life's steepest learning curves to be faced with the overwhelming love, responsibility, care and wellbeing of a new infant. Nothing compares. Knowing how, when and where to go for different aspects of parenting information and advice can provide enormous reassurance and confidence, particularly in the area of breastfeeding. As mentioned in Chapter 2, having a *resource list* that you have personally compiled before baby is born is of great value. You have the information at your fingertips for any help you need. Small concerns can become issues that can evolve into problems. It is always good to get in early with any queries you have.

I have drawn together a small list that I have found valuable and reliable over time. It is up to date as I write. The items are included only as a guide as to what may be useful for you and your family. As life unfolds with your new baby, you will be able to add to this list, and possibly share resources with others.

I emphasise the fact that no problem or issue, question or worry is too small to seek information, help or advice about. Never be afraid to ask. If not satisfied with the information you have found, try another way. There are many avenues for you to take, including books, websites, phone helplines, doctors, midwives, child health nurses, councils, and community centres. Parenting groups can be an excellent source of support and information, as can relatives and friends.

Books:

Birth With Confidence. Savvy Choices for Normal Birth, Rhea Dempsey, 2013, Griffin Press, Australia

Birth Skills. Proven Pain-management Techniques for Your Labour and Birth, Juju Sundin and Sarah Murdock, 2007, Allen and Unwin, Australia

Breastfeeding…Naturally, Australian Breastfeeding Association, 2017, Merrily Merrily Enterprises, Australia

Baby On Board, Dr Howard Chilton, 2013, Griffin Press, Australia

Breastfeeding Answers Made Simple, Nancy Mohrbacher, 2012, Hale Publishing, USA

The Ultimate Breastfeeding Book of Answers, Jack Newman & Teresa Pitman, 2006, Crown Publishing Group, USA

Breastfeeding Without Birthing, Alyssa Schnell, 2013, Praeclarus Press, USA

Mothering Multiples: Breastfeeding and Caring for Twins or More, Karen Kerkhoff Gromada, 2007, La Leche League International, USA

Defining Your Own Success. Breastfeeding After Breast Reduction Surgery, Diana West 2001, La Leche League International, USA

Baby-Led Weaning, Gill Rapley & Tracey Murkett, Ebury Publishing, UK

Breastfeeding Matters. What we need to know about infant feeding,

Maureen Minchin, 1988, Alma Publications, Australia

Help from a lactation consultant

Lactation consultants (IBCLC) are health professionals who specialise in the clinical management of breastfeeding and lactation. IBCLC's are certified by the International Board of Lactation Consultant Examiners under the direction of the US National Commission for Certifying Agencies. IBCLCs work in a variety of settings, including hospitals, pediatric offices, public health clinics and in private practice. Care is provided in your home or the consultant's office in the community.

In any country, to find a lactation consultant (FALC), go to this website and search by entering your location: www.ilca.org/why-ibclc/falc

Specific countries' Breastfeeding Helpline contacts and phone numbers:

Most countries have websites and phone numbers you can contact for help and advice.

Australia: Australian Breastfeeding Association: www.breastfeeding.asn.au National Breastfeeding Helpline—1-800-686-268

Canada: Hospital for Sick Children in Toronto: www.motherisk.org/ Motherisk Helpline—1877-439-2744

China: International Breastfeeding Party Information: www.muruhui.org/hyxx.asp

Ireland: Breastfeeding Help and Information: www.lalecheleagueireland.com

Singapore: Breastfeeding Mothers' Support Group Counselling Helpline: 63393558

United Kingdom: National Breastfeeding Helpline/Helpline: 03001000212 www.nationalbreastfeedinghelpline.org.uk/

United States of America: La Leche League USA Breastfeeding Helpline 1-877-452-5324

For any other countries: La Leche League International—Find breastfeeding help www.llli.org/get-help/

Drugs or medication and breastfeeding

Many families wonder about a particular medication that they need to take when they are breastfeeding. A good contact for this is LactMed, which is a US-based online database containing information on drugs and other chemicals to which breastfeeding mothers may be exposed: Lactmed. www.toxnet.nlm.nih.gov

Main world health authorities:

The health authorities that work together to make evidence-based recommendations for better global health and wellbeing are the World Health Organisation, *WHO,* and in Australia, The National Health and Medical Research Council, *NHMRC.* Employees work systematically to improve health outcomes in a complex and rapidly changing world by making specific recommendations for countries to follow. Significant recommendations relating to breastfeeding are:

Breastfeeding should be initiated within the first hour after birth, and exclusive breastfeeding is recommended for the first six months of age, to be continued and combined with appropriate complementary foods up to two years of age or beyond.

Another principal global health authority is the United Nations International Children's Fund, *UNICEF.* Together with the *WHO* in 1991, initiated and developed the *Baby Friendly Hospital Initiative BFHI. BFHI* is a powerful tool to encourage and enable hospital and maternity staff to achieve high levels of encouragement and support for women to breastfeed successfully. A maternity unit can be accredited as *baby friendly* when it does not accept free or low-cost milk substitutes, feeding bottles or teats and has implemented ten specific steps to support breastfeeding. Many hospitals around the world are working towards accreditation to have *BFHI* status. The growth of these hospitals is continuing to make a positive impact on breastfeeding outcomes. (Perez-Escamilla et al., 2016)

It is worth asking the question when considering booking into a hospital for the birth of your baby: *Is this hospital BFHI accredited?* If so, it would mean that you may have better breastfeeding support and encouragement in the early days when it is vital.

In 2006 *BFHI* became *'Breastfeeding Friendly Health Initiative'* in order to more accurately reflect the expansion of the initiative into the community health facilities.

WHO: www.who.int/topics/breastfeeding/en

NHMRC: www.nhmrc.gov.au/

UNICEF: www.unicef.org/

BFHI: www.unicef.org/programme/breastfeeding/baby.htm

Sites in different countries, states, cities and towns that may be useful to research for individual information and resources, could be found using similar wording as below, but making it a question relating to your specific area. For example, 'which hospitals are BFHI accredited in Adelaide, South Australia'?

BFHI accredited hospitals

Antenatal and postnatal depression services and assistance

Breastfeeding and employment—support and information

Multiple births—information and support for parents

New parent education classes—location and availability

Community Health Centres—location

Child Health Centres—location

Single parents—support and resources

Websites: There is much to be found on websites, blogs and facebook pages that is incorrect and misleading about breastfeeding, so be discerning when you choose to delve into the internet for information. When considering, look for information that is evidence-based, is nonjudgmental and offers a balanced perspective. These are a few that I have found to be reliable and where you may find useful information:

Australian Breastfeeding Association

Analytic armadillo

Best for Babes

Breastfeeder reporter

Normal, like breathing

Kellymom

The Milk Meg

The Leaky Boob

Pregnant Chicken

Hubbub The Bub Hub blog

Breastfeeding Medicine

The Academy of Breastfeeding Medicine ABM

The sceptical OB

Breastfeeding USA

Brilliant Breastfeeding: A Sensible Guide, is just that. I hope you find it helps to clear the myths and confusion that abound, and that you can simply enjoy breastfeeding your baby or babies with confidence for as long as you choose. Information in this book is supported by years of expertise, experience and evidence. Included are modern thoughts and strategies about birthing and the value of baby collecting mother's microbiome at the time of delivery. I have emphasised the importance of baby's first breastfeeds as recommended by all the world health authorities. I have also comprehensively tackled common and not so common issues that can impede breastfeeding progress.

I sincerely hope that as you are passing through this fleeting time in your life with young babies and children, you will come to know that *yes, breastfeeding is brilliant.*

References

Australian Breastfeeding Association, 2017, *Antenatal Expression of Colostrum*. Available: https://www.breastfeeding.asn.au/bfinfo/antenatal-expression-colostrum

Australian Breastfeeding Association, 2017, *Health Outcomes Associated with Infant Feeding*. Available: https://www.breastfeeding.asn.au/bfinfo/health-outcomes-associated-infant-feeding

Belford, M, July 2016, *Breastmilk Feeding, Brain Development, and Neurocognitive Outcomes: A Seven Year Longitudinal Study in Infants Born at Less than 30 weeks Gestation. The Journal of Paediatrics, DOI:10.1016/j.jpeds.2016.06.045,*

Bonyata, K, 2017, *Cluster Feeding and Fussy Evenings. Available: https://kellymom.com/parenting/parenting-faq/fussy-evening/*

Bonyata, K, 2017, *Is Your Milk Supply Really Low?* Available: www.kellymom.com

Boseley, S, 2015, *Breastfeeding. The longer babies are breastfed, the more they achieve in life—major study*. Available: https://www.theguardian.com/lifeandstyle/2015/mar/18/brazil-longer-babies-breastfed-more-achieve-in-life-major-study

Chilton, H, 2013, *Before leaping to a diagnosis*. Baby On Board, Third Edition, Griffin Press, Australia, pp. 180

Chilton, H, 2013, *Drugs in Breastmilk,* Baby On Board, Third Edition, Griffin Press, Australia, pp. 93

Chilton, H, 2013, *Giving and Receiving,* Baby On Board, Third Edition, Griffin Press, Australia, pp. 73

Chilton, H, 2013, *Sight*, Baby on Board, Third Edition, Griffin Press, Australia, pp. 111

Dahlen, H, 2018, *Birth Intervention Linked to Childhood Health Problems*, Birth, vol. 45, no. 1

Davanzo, R, 2016, *Advising Mothers on the Use of Medications During Breastfeeding: A Need for a Positive Attitude*, Journal of Human Lactation. *vol 32, Issue 1, p 15.*, vol. 32, no. 1, pp. 15

Diana Zuckerman, et al, 2018. *Are Bisphenol A (BPA) Plastic Products Safe for Infants and Children.* Available: http://www.center4research.org/bisphenol-bpa-plastic-products-safe/

Forster, D et al, 2017, Advising women with diabetes in pregnancy to express breastmilk in late pregnancy (Diabetes and Antenatal Milk Expressing [DAME]): a multicentre, unblinded, randomised controlled trial, The Lancet, vol. 389, no. 10085, pp. 2204-2213

Genna, CW & Barak, D, 2010, *Facilitating Autonomous Infant Hand Use During Breastfeeding*, Clinical Lactation, vol. 1, no. 1, pp. 15-20

Gilpin, J, 2011, *On the Breast Handbook. Planning for Breastfeeding Success*, Hyde Park Press, Australia.

Goer, H, 2017, *Laboring Down: Is it a Good Idea? Henci Goer Provides a Research Update.* Available: www.scienceandsensibility.org

Goer, H, 2017, *The Soaring Cesarean Rate: It's the Economics, Stupid.* Available: www.scienceandsensibility.org.

Gromada, K, 2007, Mothering Multiples (Too); Breastfeeding and Caring for Twins or More, Third Edition, La Leche League International, USA.

Hung, K Berg, O, 2011. *Early skin-to-skin after cesarean to improve breastfeeding*. The American Journal of Maternal/Child Nursing, 36 (5), 318-324.

Lancet Breastfeeding Series, *Key Messages and Findings*, 2017. Available: http://www.everywomaneverychild.org/wp-content/uploads/2017/02/bf3f4e_95fdf309754d

La Leche League. 2017, *Anticipating breastfeeding or now breastfeeding/expressed-breastmilk-feeding multiples: La Leche League for Mothers of Twins/ Multiples*. Available: https://www.facebook.com/groups/438068672893179/

Minchin, M, 1988, *Delayed suckling after birth*. Breastfeeding Matters. What we need to know about infant feeding. Second Edition, Alma Publications, Victoria, Australia, pp. 48.

Mohrbacher, N, 2012, *Breastfeeding and Contraception*. Breastfeeding Answers Made Simple. Pocket Guide for Helping Mothers. First Edition, Hale Publishing., Texas, USA, pp. 71-73

Mohrbacher, N, 2012, *Alcohol, Nicotine and Recreational Drugs*. Breastfeeding Answers Made Simple. A Pocket Guide for Helping Mothers. First Edition, Hale Publishing, Texas, USA, p. 214

Mohrbacher, N, 2012, *Engorgement*. Breastfeeding Answers Made Simple. A Pocket Guide for Helping Mothers, Hale Publishing, Texas USA, pp. 28

Mohrbacher, N, 2012, *Health Issues-Mother*. Breastfeeding Answers Made Simple. A Pocket Guide for Helping Mothers. First Edition, Hale Publishing, Texas, pp. 131-134

Mohrbacher, N, 2012, *Milk Production*. Breastfeeding Answers Made Simple, First Edition, Hale Publishing, Texas. USA, pp. 163.

Mohrbacher, N, 2012, *Relactation and Induced Lactation* in Breastfeeding Answers Made Simple. A Pocket Guide for Helping Mothers. First Edition, Hale Publishing, USA, pp. 239-247

Montagu, A, 1979, *Touching: The Human Significance of the Skin.* Second Edition. Harper and Row Publishing, Australia.

Newman, J & Pitman, T, 2006, *Special Situations: Adoption, Breast Surgeries, Relactation.* The Ultimate Breastfeeding Book of Answers. Three Rivers Press, USA, pp. 255-260

Newman, J & Pitman, T, 2006, *Not Enough Milk.* The Ultimate Breastfeeding Book of Answers. Three Rivers Press, USA, pp. 63-99

Palmer, B, 1998, *The Influence of Breastfeeding on the Development of the Oral Cavity*, Journal of Human Lactation. *Vol 14, Issue 2, pp 93-98.*

Pearson-Glaze, P, 2018, *Expression of Colostrum Antenatally.* Breastfeeding Support. Available: http://breastfeeding.support/expressing-colostrum-antenatally/.

Perez-Escamilla, R, Martinez, J & Segura- Perez, S, 2016, *"Impact of the Baby Friendly Initiative on Breastfeeding and Child Health Outcomes"*, Maternity and Child Nutrition, vol. 12, no. 3

Porteus, J, 2014, *What is a Baby's Microbiome and Why Should Expectant Mothers Care?* Available: http://www.healthygutbugs.com/babys-microbiome-expectant-mothers-care/.

Randle, S, 2015, *Sowing the Seeds of Future Health*. Available: http://www.imuk.org.uk/51334/.

Richardson, H, Walker, A & Horne, R, 2010, *Influence of swaddling experience on spontaneous arousal patterns and autonomic control in sleeping infants.*, J Pediatr., vol. 157, no. 1, pp. 85-91

Riordan, J & Wambach, K, 2010, *Breastfeeding and Human Lactation.* Breastfeeding and Human Lactation, Fourth Edition, Jones and Bartlett, Canada, pp. 520

Riordan, J & Wambach, K, 2010. *Postpartum depression.* Breastfeeding and Human Lactation, Fourth Edition, Jones and Bartlett, Canada, pp. 539-542

Riordan, J & Wambach, K, 2009, *Multiple Infants.* Breastfeeding and Human Lactation, Fourth Edition, Jones and Bartlett, Canada, UK, pp. 276

Savino, F, Stefania, A, Liguori, M, Fissore, F, Oggero, R, 2009, *Breastfeeding Hormones and Their Protective Effect on Obesity.* International Journal of Paediatric Endocrinology, vol. Article ID 327505

Schnell, A, 2013, *Approaches to Inducing Lactation.* Breastfeeding Without Birthing, First Edition, Praeclarus Press, Texas, USA, pp. 137-152

Schnell, A, 2013. Breastfeeding Without Birthing. A Breastfeeding Guide for Mothers through Adoption, Surrogacy and Other Special Circumstances., First Edition, Praeclarus Press, Texas, USA

Sears, D, 2018, *Breastfeeding and Brain Development. The Link Between Breastfeeding and Brain Development.* Available: https://www.askdrsears.com/topics/feeding-eating/breastfeeding/why-breast-is-best/breastfeeding-brain-development

Smith, M & Segal, J, 2018, *Postpartum Depression and the Baby Blues. Signs, Symptoms, Coping Tips and Treatment.* Available: https://www.helpguide.org/articles/depression/postpartum-depression-and-the-baby-blues.htm?pdf=true

Taskforce on SIDS, 2016. *SIDS and Other Sleep-Related Infant Deaths. Recommendations for a Safe Infant Environment.* American Academy of Pediatrics, vol. 138, no. 5, p. 2016-2938

United Nations International Children's Fund & World Health Organisation. 2017. *The Baby-Friendly Hospital Initiative. The Ten Steps to Successful Breastfeeding.* Available: https://www.unicef.org/programme/breastfeeding/baby.htm#10

West, D, 2001, Defining Your Own Success. Breastfeeding After Breast Reduction Surgery. First Edition, La Leche League International, Schaumburg, Illinois, USA

WHO, TS, 2014, *Exclusive breastfeeding to reduce the risk of childhood overweight and obesity. Biological, behavioural and contextual rationale,* e-Library of Evidence for Nutrition Actions (eLENA)

WHO, TS, 1985, *"Appropriate Technology for Birth.", Lancet,* vol. 2, no. August, pp. 436-437

Widstrom, A. & Hanson, L. 2011, *The Magical Hour. Healthy Children Project.* Available: http://www.magicalhour.org/aboutus.html.

Wikipedia 2017, *Baby Friendly Hospital Initiative.* Available: https://en.wikipedia.org/wiki/Baby_Friendly_Hospital_Initiative

Young, J, Kearney, L, Rutherford, C, Cowan, SG & K, Hoey, J, 2017, *Enabling Safe and Close Care in Postnatal Environments. (ESCCaPE Trial)* Available: http://www.anzctr.org.au/ AnzctrAttachments/373027-ESCCaPE_Protocol_CLEAN_ V1.1_20170505.pdf

Zuckerman, D & Brown, P, 2015, *Are Bisphenol A (BPA) Plastic Products Safe?* Available: http://www.center4research.org/ bisphenol-bpa-plastic-products-safe/

Acknowledgements

I could not have written this book without the parents who were willing to share their intimate birth and breastfeeding photographs and experiences. I whole-heartedly thank them.

Jo, Azlin and Indra

Airlie, Michael, Lachie and Alice

Anna, Alex and Lucy

Robbie, Lisa and Delilah

Lissy, Nikki, Indy and Ari

Airlie, Tom and Winston

Holly, Ed and Evander

Laura, Pete and Pippi

Helen, Joey and Frankie

Nick, Bec and Finlay

These parents, and others, with whom I have been privileged to work with, firm my belief that breastfeeding can be made easier with thoughtful preparation, evidence-based information and encouragement. It is every mother's right to be supported to breastfeed her babies if she chooses. And every baby's right to receive breastmilk whenever possible.

I acknowledge the excellent work of midwives, dedicated lactation consultant colleagues, global health organisations and some governments that work towards the aim of raising world breastfeeding statistics. When mothers breastfeed and babies are breastfed with confidence, we all win!

I sincerely thank my editor Jude Aquilina, Gary MacRae from solopublishing for his formatting work and the staff at South Australia's Open Book Howden, for finalising this book. I also thank my friend Jennie Teasdale, who has shown consistent mentor ship and encouragement for me to complete this project, as have my husband and children.

Jo Gilpin, 2018

Index

Formula 23-24

Foremilk 129

Freezing of breastmilk 188-190

Frenotomy 100-101

Finger-feeding 109, 110

Foods beside breastmilk 149-157

Frenulum *see* Tongue-tie 100

Fruit juice 155

Fertility 142

G

Gag reflex 154

Galactagogues 115

Gastro-oesophageal reflux *see*
    Reflux 126-128

Gestational diabetes 31-32, 47-48

Growth charts 89

Growth surges 91

H

Hand expression of
    breastmilk 106-107

Hindmilk 129

Home birth 49-50, 64

Hormones 12

I

Increasing milk Supply 115-118

Intelligence 22

J

Jaundice 31, 94

K

'Kangaroo-care' 63

L

Lactose intolerance 130

Leptin 22

Let-down reflex 16

Low Supply 115-119

M

Mastitis 122-126, 188, 200

Meconium 73-74, 94

Medications *see* Drugs

Menstruation 85-86, 137, 204

N

Natural senses 52, 60

Night feeds 84-86, 160-168

Nipple confusion 39, 100

Nipple shields 104-105

O

Obesity 22, 152-153, 194

Oral Thrush 101-102

Overabundant milk supply 120-122

Oxytocin 12, 16, 19-20, 86, 114,
    132, 186-187

P

Pacifiers (dummies) 75-76

Partial breastfeeding 199-200

Phototherapy 94

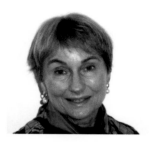

Jo Gilpin has worked with parents and their babies for over thirty years. She is the mother of three breastfed children, a registered midwife, child and family health nurse and lactation consultant.

Jo is a member of ILCA and LCANZ, and keeps in constant touch with lactation consultant colleagues. *Brilliant Breastfeeding: A Sensible Guide* is Jo's second book. The first, printed in 2011 was *On the Breast Handbook: Planning for Breastfeeding Success.*

Jo now lives and continues her work in a private practice on Kangaroo Island, South Australia.